TRANSACTIONS

OF THE

AMERICAN PHILOSOPHICAL SOCIETY

HELD AT PHILADELPHIA
FOR PROMOTING USEFUL KNOWLEDGE

———

NEW SERIES—VOLUME 61, PART 3
1971

———

PRACTICAL OBSERVATIONS ON DROPSY OF THE CHEST (BRESLAU, 1706)

Translated and Edited by
SAUL JARCHO, M.D.

———

THE AMERICAN PHILOSOPHICAL SOCIETY
INDEPENDENCE SQUARE
PHILADELPHIA

MARCH, 1971

This publication is based on research assisted by the National Institutes of Health (HE–10948). The author is indebted to the National Library of Medicine and the library of the New York Academy of Medicine, as well as to Mrs. Richard North and Miss Françoise Duvivier, for assistance given during various parts of the study.

PRACTICAL OBSERVATIONS ON DROPSY OF THE CHEST (BRESLAU, 1706)

Translated and edited by

SAUL JARCHO, M.D.

CONTENTS

INTRODUCTION

In the year 1705, Leopold I, Holy Roman Emperor and king of Bohemia and Hungary, died of dropsy of the chest (hydrothorax). His loyal subjects, the members of the Leopoldine Academy of Scientists, a group which he had honored and protected, resolved to commemorate his eventful reign by preparing an essay on the disease that had caused his death. The treatise was published in 1706 at Breslau in a quarto volume of sixty-two pages titled *Observationes Practicae de Hydrope Pectoris, in Quibus de Signis et Causis Occultioris Hujus Morbi, ac Curandi Ratione Disseritur, a Colleg. Acad. Leopold. Nat. Curios. Vratislaviens. Editae* (Practical Observations on Dropsy of the Chest, in Which the Signs, Causes, and Method of Treatment of this Very Obscure Disease are Discussed; Issued by the Leopoldine Academy of Scientists at Breslau).[1]

The Leopoldine Academy was founded by Dr. Johann Lorenz Bausch of Schweinfurt, who invited three colleagues to an initial meeting, which took place in that city of January 1, 1652. At first the organization was named Academia Naturae Curiosorum. Its sphere of interest was defined as medicine and the natural sciences related to medicine.

The earliest activities of the Academy are largely unrecorded. Apparently the organization had no fixed site; it migrated—with its growing library—to the various cities of successive presidents until 1878, when Halle was chosen as the permanent location. The Academy celebrated its tercentenary in 1952 and is now well into its fourth century.

The activities of the academicians were of course not limited to the Academy or to the clinical aspects of medicine and the Academy's publication, the *Ephemerides*. For example, an academician and clergyman named Caspar Neumann (1648–1715) compiled the vital statistics of Breslau for the years 1687–1691. Through the agency of Henri Justell, secretary of the Royal Society of London, these tabulations reached Edmund Halley, the English astronomer, who used them to compile his famous *Estimate of the Degrees of Mortality of Mankind . . . with an Attempt to Ascertain the Price of Annuities upon Lives.*[2]

Unlike its seventeenth-century contemporaries, the Academy did not hold sessions at which experiments were demonstrated. Its chief activities were discussion and publication. Its official periodical, the *Ephemerides Naturae Curiosorum*, came into existence in 1670 and has had several changes of name, the most recent instar being designated *Nova Acta Leopoldina*. This periodical continues to be issued.[3]

The treatise which is here under consideration was issued as a separate volume and not as part of the *Ephemerides*. Since the title page states that the book was issued *a Colleg. Acad. Leopold. Nat. Curios. Vratislaviens.*, the expressions "Breslau authors" and "Breslau physicians" have been devised for collective reference in the present analysis; it is not intended to imply that all the anonymous authors of the book necessarily resided at Breslau. The confusing Latin terms *Vratislava* and *Vratislaviensis* refer to Breslau and not to the city of Bratislava, which is situated in Slovakia and was formerly called Pressburg.

Evidence is extant which suggests that at least part of the text—and possibly the whole of it—was composed by Christianus Helwich (1666–1770). In his essay *Observata quaedam ex anatome matronae difficiliori respiratione per totum vitae spatium laborantis* (Observations made at the autopsy of a woman who had suffered from lifelong difficulty of respiration), published in the *Ephemerides*, centuria 10, observatio 32, pp. 307–310, 1722,[4] Helwich tells of a pathognomonic clinical sign "which was established by

---

[1] I have used a photocopy made available through the courtesy of the National Library of Medicine.

[2] *Phil. Trans.* 17 (1693): pp. 23–28. London, 1694; addendum, pp. 654–656. See also Lowell J. Reed, editor, *Degrees of Mortality of Mankind by Edmund Halley as Presented in his Papers* (Baltimore, 1942). See also Jonas Graetzer, *Edmund Halley und Caspar Neumann* (Breslau, 1883).

[3] Andreas Büchner, *Academiae Sacri Romani Imperii Leopoldinae Naturae Curiosorum Historia* (Magdeburg, 1755). Rudolph Zaunick, "Dreihundert Jahre Leopoldina," *Nova Acta Leopoldina* 15 (1952): pp. 31–42. Martha Ornstein, *The Role of Scientific Societies in the Seventeenth Century* (3d ed., reprinted, New York, 1963), pp. 169–175.

[4] English translation in Saul Jarcho, "Christianus Helwich on Difficulty of Respiration (Augsburg, 1722)," *Bull. N. Y. Acad. Med.* 46 (1970): pp. 34–38.

3

Carolus Piso ... and which is repeated by me in *Practical Observations on Dropsy of the Chest*, published in the name of the Academy of Sciences at Breslau." Hence Helwich must have done the actual writing of at least a portion of the text, although it is clear that other physicians were consulted. Possibly the different chapters or sections were prepared by different academicians.

According to an official history of the academy,[5] Helwich was adviser and archiater to several nobles and magnates of Silesia and municipal physician at Breslau. He was born in Prussia on June 25, 1666. He was admitted to the academy in 1695 and died in Breslau on September 20, 1740. The index to the third *decuria* of the *Ephemerides*,[6] which covers the period from 1693 to 1706, lists no less than thirty-nine papers credited to Helwich. These deal with what might be called miscellaneous clinical subjects such as smallpox, menstrual disorders, calculi, gangrene, tabes, parotitis, and other conditions.

The Breslau volume is a thorough, systematic monograph, adequately detailed and relatively clear. It was prepared by, or under the aegis of, a group of leading practitioners and professors. For these reasons it is an instructive indicator of the condition of medical thought and practice in the early eighteenth century. Moreover, despite the plethora of technical detail that it necessarily provides and despite the impersonal character to be expected in a treatise which was prepared under the auspices of a committee and bears the name of no individual author, it does not completely conceal the distinctive traits of the practicing physician; these peep out from time to time in the discussion.

But the Breslau treatise provides more than a general indication of the state of medicine in 1706. In dealing with hydrothorax, it exhibits in detail the condition of cardiology at a point in time almost exactly equidistant between Harvey's *De Motu Cordis* (1628) and Withering's *Account of the Foxglove* (1785). In this respect the salient feature is the failure to recognize heart disease as a cause of hydrothorax.

The book opens with a grandiloquent dedicatory address to the Emperor Joseph I, successor to Leopold I. While the obsequious tone of this exordium is repellent to today's taste, it reminds the modern reader of the dependence of the eighteenth-century physician and scientist on the patronage of royalty and nobility. Such dependence on governmental power may be compared with phenomena of the contemporary scene.

The second preface, addressed to the reader, opens with Baglivi's admonition concerning the establishment of learned societies. Baglivi's advice had failed of acceptance in Germany, in part because of an almost epidemic contempt for older medical doctrines. This malady, however, did not affect all physicians; and Germany had always had outstanding men who took exact account of what had been written in any era about any given disease, its course, and treatment, and compared these records with their own observations.

A similar procedure was adopted by the Breslau authors in the present treatise. Considering their personal experience inadequate for the preparation of a complete study, they freely consulted the writings of others. This involved them in the problem of citation, and their difficulties are significant of the condition of bibliographic technique in 1706.

Avoiding recourse to footnotes and marginalia, they use simple reference citation incorporated in the text and followed by verbatim quotation in italics.[7] The references usually give the author's name and the exact or approximate title of the book, followed by the section number, chapter number, and page number, *but not the place or date of publication*. In other words, the reader is informed that the passage quoted occurred in book so-and-so, in chapter so-and-so, and on page so-and-so, but he is not told which edition was used. Here are three examples:

... apud Tulpium *l. 2. Observ. c. 16. p. 128* ...

Hippocrates *lib. 2 de morb. n. 59. p.m. 84. tom. 2.* ait ...

Carolus Piso in *selectis suis Observ. & Consilis de praetervisis hactenus morbis à serosa colluvie ortis, sect. 3. cap. 7. p. 296.* his verbis ...

In these specimens the quotation from Tulpius is readily recognized as having been taken from the edition of the *Observationes Medicae* published by Elzevier in Amsterdam in 1652. The passage from Hippocrates corresponds in pagination with the edition of van der Linden, Leyden, 1665; for the convenience of the modern reader I have regularly added to each Hippocratic citation a footnote containing the page number in the more convenient edition of C. G. Kühn, Leipzig, 1825–1827.

With respect to the passage taken from Piso the page numbers show that the Breslau academicians did not use the edition published by Mercator at Pont-à-Mousson in 1618, nor was I able to determine which edition they did use. Hence I have footnoted all citations of Piso by reference to the accessible Leyden 1714 edition, although it is later than our

---

[5] Andreas Büchner, *op. cit.* ref. 3, p. 481. See also Jonas Graetzer, *Lebensbilder Hervorragender Schlesischer Aerzte* (Breslau, 1889), p. 209.

[6] *Index Generalis et Absolutissimus Decuriae Tertiae Ephemeridum* . . . (Frankfurt, 1713).

[7] In translating the quotations I have disregarded the italics. In some instances a quotation is followed by the enigmatic abbreviation *H. I.* From another of the Academy's publications, the *Historia morborum qui annis mdcic, mdcc, mdcci, Vratislaviae grassati sunt* (Breslau and Leipzig, Banckius, 1706) it is deduced that this stands for *hactenus ille*, which is roughly equivalent to "end of quotation."

Breslau treatise. A similar procedure has been necessary with several other authors, in whom I have had to be content with verifying the passage without always being able to find the same edition that was consulted by the scholars of Breslau.

These bibliographic difficulties suggest that in presenting quotations and references the Breslau academicians were interested mainly in avoiding misstatement and in preventing accusations of plagiarism, whereas the modern scholar compiles references to facilitate independent verification by the reader and to demonstrate that primary sources have been consulted.

THE NATURAL HISTORY OF THE DISEASE

The text proper of the *De Hydrope Pectoris* is divided into three chapters, which deal respectively with the natural history of the malady, its causes, and its treatment. Let us consider these components in turn.

The chapter devoted to natural history covers both clinical course and anatomical findings. Pectoral dropsy, say the Breslau authors, is usually not recognized while the patient is alive. It is usually preceded by oppression and discomfort about the precordia (I. 2).[8] Similar symptoms also precede ascites. The oppression and discomfort do not always make the physician able to conjecture that pectoral dropsy impends.

Severe respiratory difficulty occurs in pectoral dropsy and also in ascites, in asthma, and in some other diseases of the chest (I. 3). According to Hippocrates, persons afflicted with these conditions have a rapid difficult respiration and appear to be suffocating. This does not occur in wet asthma, the distinctive sign of which is a loud whistling noise and a bubbling sound. Hoarseness occurs in asthma but not in hydrothorax. Further, an asthmatic can hold his breath for a long time; persons afflicted with pectoral dropsy cannot do this but it is not certain that the criterion is infallible.

Pectoral dropsy characteristically awakens the patient after he has had a few hours of sleep and it remits as dawn approaches (I. 3). Carolus Piso called this a pathognomonic sign and Lazarus Riverius agreed. Bonetus however reported a four-pound collection of fluid in a maiden who had had neither dyspnoea nor orthopnoea; such cases must be considered very rare. The experience of the Breslau academicians supports the opinion of Piso.

The literature reports various kinds of pulse (I. 4) in pectoral dropsy, especially intermittent pulse. Very recently Dr. Helwich recognized the disease in a man who had presented this irregularity. The diagnosis of pectoral dropsy was confirmed at autopsy.

In addition to palpitation (I. 5) and fainting, the patients have symptoms (I. 6) that are caused by the massiveness of the fluid, which presses the diaphragm down. There is difficulty in breathing when the body must be moved and pain is felt in the back over the attachments of the diaphragm. The water may be felt to fluctuate or move about when the body is bent, and direct auscultation may be attempted after the method of Hippocrates, confirmed by Zacutus Lusitanus.

The more accurate differentiation between hydrothorax and empyema (I. 6) depends on the history of antecedent illnesses such as whooping cough, pleuritis, and pneumonia and also on examination for the presence of such signs as sweating, contracted nostrils, flushed face, and warm palms and soles. If these signs are absent, the sensation of fluid moving in the chest indicates that hydrothorax is present.

Other signs are dry cough (I. 7) and swelling of the genitalia (I. 8). The genitals may swell earlier than the feet or the abdomen. The swelling of the feet usually starts near the malleoli. While the abdomen is filling, the patient's symptoms may remit and he may congratulate himself on a false improvement. The upper extremities may become thin while the lower extremities swell (I. 9).

The next symptom to be considered is fever. The extended discussion of fever in hydrothorax (I. 10) might almost be taken independently as an indicator of the condition of medical knowledge and thought in 1706. The passage begins, in the customary way, with a consideration of Hippocratic statements, but shows scholarly skepticism as to the genuineness of the ancient text. "The author of the book *De Morbis*, which goes under the name of Hippocrates" puts fever first among the signs of hydrothorax. The Breslau authors have learned from experience that fever and hydrothorax occasionally coexist. Confirmatory evidence was reported by Fonseca, Piso, Coiter, Chesneau, and Pompeius Saccus.

It is instructive to examine some of the original reports on which these references were based. Fonseca's patient,[9] a man aged forty, had had two years of severe respiratory difficulty and dry cough. The hypochondria, scrotum, feet, and eyelids were swollen. Low fever was present and some of the traditional Hippocratic observations—as puzzling in Fonseca as in Hippocrates—were made, i.e., a sound resembling the fluctuation of water was perceived when the patient was turned to either side, and on direct auscultation a noise like that of vinegar (ebullition?) was heard. The pulses were very uneven. The outcome is not stated but the modern reader finds no great difficulty in accepting the case as one of hydrothorax or perhaps hydropneumothorax.

---

[8] References will be made to chapter and section of the Breslau text. In this instance the reference is to chapter 1, section 2.

[9] Rodericus à Fonseca, *Consultationes Medicae* (Venice, 1619–1622), consult. 54, 1: p. 197.

Piso's patient,[10] a sixty-year old canon, had fever and "catarrh in the chest" and was sick for six weeks. After an interval of good health he was taken with a prolonged chill, accompanied by fever and severe dyspnoea and orthopnoea. He had conspicuous swelling of both hypochondria, especially the right. Autopsy revealed a greatly enlarged hard liver, and a huge quantity of clear fluid in the chest. The duration of the final illness is not stated. The onset with prolonged chill suggests that the case may have been one of pneumonia, which was followed by heart failure.

The case of Nicolaus Chesneau[11] was quite obviously one of puerperal sepsis and suppurative pneumonitis and pleuritis; this requires no extended commentary. The case of Pompeius Saccus[12] concerned an alcoholic surgeon who had felt water moving within his body. This report is rather unclear. Possibly the patient suffered from cirrhosis of the liver with ascites and hydrothorax, in addition to fever.

These examples show that most of the cases which the Breslau authors selected from the literature would probably satisfy modern criteria of hydrothorax. It is equally evident that these cases were of widely diverse etiology and that the state of medical knowledge did not make possible a satisfactory etiological classification.

Having presented a sample of reported cases in which hydrothorax was accompanied by fever, the authors significantly add: "Indeed, others suffering from this kind of dropsy are free from fever, as we have noticed time and again." This statement of first-hand experience is then corroborated by additional citations from the literature.

It is not surprising that the Breslau academicians were widely read. Their citations extend over the whole of the literature then available but are not excessively numerous and appear to have been well chosen; no attempt was made to impress the reader by a profusion of references. The passages which they selected for citation or quotation were often judged carefully and were almost always tested against the personal experiences of the academicians. On the specific instance at hand they concluded that fever occasionally occurs in hydrothorax but that this conjunction was by no means invariable.

Continuing their catalog of symptoms, the Breslau authors briefly mention pain and paralysis in the arms, susceptibility to cold, and haemoptysis (I. 11). Paralysis of the arms accompanying hydrothorax does

not correspond to anything recognized nowadays in ordinary clinical experience; hence the statement is a minor historical enigma, worthy of separate study. The symptom is discussed again in the chapter on causes (II. 19). Other interesting clinical observations are the tendency of patients to become "asthmatic," i.e. dyspnoeic, after a large meal (I. 12); the occurrence of profuse micturition *before* a paroxysm (I. 13) of dyspnoea; and the tendency of the disease to end suddenly after a protracted course (I. 14).

In the presentation of the autopsy findings priority is given to descriptions of the fluid (I. 15). As might be expected, a great variety of colors and qualities is reported, including clear, citrinous, mucinous, bloody, purulent, caseous, and fetid. An especially confusing variety is that found in hydatid cysts, which remained a stumbling-block to pathology for many years. The variety of the fluids mentioned in this part of the text showed that the scope included almost all the etiological types known to us.

Similar diversity was apparent in the lungs of hydropic persons (I. 17), according to cases which the Breslau academicians collected from the literature. Scirrhi, tubercles, hydatids, purulent and putrid changes, and gangrene were reported in cases of hydrothorax.

Various types of pericardial change were found also. These include fleshy thickening, lentil-sized granules, and reddish speckling. In one published case the aorta was roughened and ossified near the semilunar valves. These few comments include *all* that the Breslau scholars collected as to anatomical changes in the hearts of persons afflicted with hydrothorax. Nothing is said about the myocardium, the valves, or the coronary vessels. Alterations in other organs (I. 17) include hardening and swelling of the liver, enlargement of the spleen, and ulceration and suppuration of the kidneys.

A special section (I. 18) is devoted to the condition of the glands in dropsical persons. The discussion deals entirely with a case published by Otto Heurnius, who had found hydrothorax and ascites in a fourteen-year-old girl. The collections of fluid were accompanied by universal enlargement of glands. The liver, spleen, and lung were bestrewn as if by hail. This report, representing perhaps miliary tuberculosis or lymphoma, is offered without further comment as an indication of the behavior of the glands in hydrothorax. It is not clear why this single case was considered so important and it is equally unclear why no comment was appended to it.

THE CAUSES OF PECTORAL DROPSY

The second chapter of the Breslau treatise is titled *The Causes of Dropsy of the Chest* and is divided into twenty sections. Only the most significant and interesting will be reviewed here.

[10] Carolus Piso, *Selectiorum Observationum et Consiliorum de Praetervisis Hactenus Morbis Affectionisbusque Praeter Naturam ab Aqua seu Serosa Colluvie et Diluvie Ortis* (Leyden, 1714), sect. 3, chap. 7, obs. 54, pp. 239–240.

[11] Nicolas Chesneau, *Observationum Medicarum Libri Quinque* (Leyden, 1719), book 5, obs. 9, pp. 480–487.

[12] Pompeius Saccus, *Medicina Theorico-Practica* (Parma, 1687), pp. 114 and 107–109.

The authors commence their consideration of etiology by attempting to discover the anatomical sources of the fluid. They take up first the contention of Willis (II. 1), who had assumed that the blood boils or bubbles in the precordia. When the resultant vapors are denied free egress, they condense and accumulate. The process was envisioned as a sort of distillation, such as might take place in an alembic. Our commentators reject this hypothesis on the ground that if it were true, all animals that breathe and have vigorous circulation would suffer frequently from hydrothorax.

It is interesting to observe that refutation of the Willisian hypothesis was accomplished by reasoning and not by recourse to observation. A modern physiologist or physician would simply have pointed out that no one had ever seen blood boiling in the precordium.

Since no fluid comes down into the thorax from the head (II. 2), and any pathways which might lead into the chest from the liver and spleen are involved in total obscurity, it is necessary to conclude that serous fluid enters the chest from opened and disrupted vessels in the thorax. Indeed such anatomists as Pecquetus, Nuck, and Malpighi had demonstrated a great profusion of lymphatics in the chest. Moreover (II. 3) the old belief in the existence of a nerve fluid is not supported by most of the recent anatomical researches. "Therefore it must be that the serous fluid is poured out into the cavity of the chest either from the blood vessels, the lymphatics, or both."

The physical appearance of lymph (II. 4) shows it to be the same as thoracic fluid. If lymphatic vessels are damaged or obstructed, lymph enters the pleural cavity; it may also enter the thoracic cavity from broken glands, as is shown by Bartholinus' case[13] of hydatid disease. Further confirmation is obtained from a case of hydrothorax reported by Willis,[14] whose patient had the sensation of a vessel bursting in his chest and then felt a dripping of fluid in the thoracic cavity.

Willis reached the not unreasonable opinion (II. 5) that weak and watery blood exudes excess serum from the vessels into the thoracic cavity. The Breslau authors agree. In addition they had observed that uninjured blood vessels in the subcutaneous tissues were sometimes opened by their own weakness and by the weakness of the blood. This opinion they bolster by the analogy of hydrocephalus.

At this point the modern reader may feel inclined to pause and wonder at the fact that contemporary doctrines of transudation had been so closely approached by the Breslau physicians and their immediate predecessors, who used ratiocination and

analogy and lacked any significant amount of really demonstrative evidence.

Continuing, the authors point out (II. 5) that the occasional presence of admixed blood is further evidence that thoracic fluid is of intravascular origin. However, despite all these considerations, it must be confessed that the manner of outflow of serum from blood vessels and lymphatics cannot be determined accurately and is not of much importance to the practitioner. The existence of urine, tears, sweat, catarrh, and diarrhoea shows how readily serum is separated from blood.

The cause of the extravasation of lymph and serum (II. 7) must be sought in the fluids, or the vessels and viscera, or in all together.

The effusion of lymph is considered first. Here the reader comes upon an elaborate pathogenesis which seems almost wholly imaginary and which contrasts with some of the common-sense remarks already discussed.

Thickness of the lymph (II. 7) prevents resorption and causes obstruction. Inspissated lymph overpowers the delicate pores and channels, and by humidity weakens them and disposes them to rupture. Through stasis the lymph becomes acrid and salty. It may become mucoid when not separated properly from salty and fatty serum which abounds in mucoid elements; such separation should occur in the liver and the impairment of separation likewise occurs especially in the liver. Hence diseased livers are found post mortem in cases of ascites and hydrothorax. Consequently it is not illogical to look in the abdomen for the cause of effusions in the chest.

The disease is aggravated when the serum affected by mucoid dyscrasia is not cleared by transpiration or urination. The lymph is thickened by cold drinks taken in hot weather, by cold air, and by aqua vitae. The effect of alcohol was demonstrated experimentally by Boyle (II. 7), who showed that spirit mixed with blood causes the latter to coagulate.

Diseases of vessels (II. 8) must also be considered as possible causes of hydrothorax but at present none are known except narrowness and laxity. Narrowness may be due to abnormal conformation at birth, or to pressure from inflammations or scirrhi, or to astringent medications. It is well known that suppression of fever by an astringent medicine leads to dropsy. The same happens after excessively energetic treatment of nosebleed.

Dropsy due to disease of vessels becomes worse rapidly and is hard to cure. Disease of vessels is often combined with disease of viscera, especially of the lungs, which may be affected by hardness, scirrhosity, swelling, and cavitation. Pleural adhesions obstruct the flow of lymph but do not immediately cause pectoral dropsy.

How does it happen (II. 9) that the blood sends out its serum from its vessels and into the cavity of

---

[13] Thomas Bartholinus, *Historiarum Anatomicarum Rariorum Centuria I et II* (Amsterdam, 1654), centuria 2, historia 66, p. 263.

[14] Thomas Willis, *Pharmaceutice Rationalis, Pars Secunda* (London, 1675), sect. 1, chap. 13, p. 229.

the chest? As was stated previously (II. 7), we must recognize that disease may be present in the blood, or in the vessels and viscera, or in both.

Although acrimony and salinity of the blood are injurious, the main cause of trouble is viscidity, which produces obstruction. The viscidity comes from "dyspepsia" (bad cooking) or inadequate conversion of crude and inert substances. Other causes are a transfer of dregs to the blood. The result is stagnation and inflammation in viscera.

It is most important that impeded lymphatic flow and the outpouring of lymph into any cavity greatly increase the viscidity of the blood and favor stagnation in vessels. It is known by reason and experience that venous blood is ten times thicker than arterial, whereas arterial blood contains ten times more lymph than does venous blood. Venous blood requires dilution in order to flow back to the heart, and God has provided abundant lymphatic vessels for this purpose. If the movement of lymph is delayed or the lymph has been effused into a cavity and has failed to enter the venous blood, the latter will fail to become diluted and will be abnormally thick. In consequence stagnation and obstruction will arise.

When blood vessels are compressed, serum pours forth separately from blood; this was shown by Lower's experimental vascular ligations.

Effusion of serum thus results from a combination of viscidity of the blood and disease of blood vessels and lymphatic vessels. In consequence of these changes the vessels and viscera become stuffed with glutinous blood. These effects are illustrated by the report of Blanckard.[16] He found coagula at the root of the aorta; these had caused deficiencies in the pulse.

"Ossification" (calcification) of arteries (II. 10) also participates in the process by delaying the movement of the blood and favoring stagnation. This is shown in the autopsy of the famous Wepfer. His blood had been dashed against bony arterial irregularities and lymph flowed out into the chest. Similar effects can be produced by polypous intravascular concretions (II. 10).

The statement about polypous concretions requires brief comment. These concretions, now known to be postmortem clots, were for many years a stumbling block to pathology. The fact that they were sometimes found in cases of hydrothorax was a misleading coincidence from which medical science could not be liberated until a greater quantity of anatomical experience had accumulated.

In attempting to explain hydrothorax the Breslau academicians could not ignore pericardial dropsy (II. 12). They state at first that it arises in the same way as pleural dropsy, except that the move-

ment of the heart plays a larger role. They recognize that fluid in the pericardial cavity impedes filling of the heart, since "the heart cannot dilate sufficiently to take up [incoming] blood." Having come this far they then negate the discussion of etiology by adding "no one expects from us that we should decide whether water drips from the pericardium into the chest through concealed ducts or goes frequently from the chest into the pericardium, although the first of these opinions appears to us to be by far the most likely."

Of the visceral "defects," i.e., lesions (II. 13), that accompany pectoral dropsy, some are causes and some are consequences. Causes include, vaguely, "the more important diseases of the filtering organs and various corruptions of the liver, spleen, lungs, etc." The renal diseases are a result. The reader is not told how the differentiation between causes and results was made. Nothing is said about heart disease as a possible cause. Diseases of the lungs "participate in the generation of this disease more effectively than diseases of other organs ..." (II. 13) and dropsy of the chest is quite well known in that time of life in which congestions in the chest are common. Remoter causes of pectoral dropsy (II. 14) are enumerated without proof or evidence and include coarse food, unsuitable drink, bad air, idleness, and emotion. Pectoral dropsy is said to follow scurvy, asthma, dysentery, and hemoptysis.

Although they had decided to devote Chapter II of their treatise to the causes of pectoral dropsy, the Breslau authors now revert to the symptoms (II. 15). Apparently they felt that a consideration of cause must embrace not only the causes of the disease but also the cause of each symptom. The first to be considered is pain.

Precordial pain (II. 15) is an indication that fluid is held outside vessels and causes distention of fibers. Tension can be produced even by very small amounts of fluid. This is proved in a curious way: persons who suffer from ascites may have pain in the feet even when no noteworthy swelling is present.

A most important discussion (II. 15) concerns a major symptom of pectoral dropsy, viz. attacks of suffocation occurring after the first period of sleep. How can this conspicuous phenomenon be explained? Willis attributed it to vapors which arise because of the warmth of sleep. The Breslau physicians find that the nocturnal "asthma" occurs usually five hours after dinner. At this time the stomach has been empty for one hour but chyle has not fully entered the lacteal vessels. The nocturnal restlessness can therefore be ascribed to chyle flowing into the bloodstream but not yet properly mixed with it. At this point in the discussion, as at many other junctures, the modern reader cannot help noticing the importance which the Breslau academicians ascribe to lymphatics in the causation of disease. It is quite evident that

16 Stephanus Blanckard, *Anatomia Practica Rationalis* (Amsterdam, 1688), centuria 2, obs. 48, p. 265.

the anatomical discoveries of the preceding century had made a very great impression and had tilted physiological concepts to an extent not supported by available evidence.

In sleep, say our authors (II. 15), not only the muscles but also the vessels and the glands are relaxed. Hence there is increased afflux of fluid to the chest, with greater compression of the lungs and greater interruption of breathing.

Since irregularity and intermittence of the pulse (II. 16) were considered symptomatic of hydrothorax, these epiphenomena were felt to require explanation. They were attributed to an impediment in the disturbances in blood flow. The pulse is equal when blood is expelled into the arteries in equal quantities and with equal force during equal intervals of time. Inequality of the pulse is therefore due to delay within the heart or to impediment in the influx or efflux of blood or other fluids. Weakness and intermittence of the pulse can also be caused by an agglomeration of thick fluid which envelops the ventricles and the blood vessels; this dictum was taken, without critical analysis, from Lower.

Fainting (II. 17) is due to temporary obstruction in large blood vessels near the heart. Patients who faint often are likely to die suddenly. Cough (II. 18) is caused by sharp fluid that irritates the diaphragm, lungs, and larynx; as the fluid ferments the irritation increases. Fever (II. 19) does not arise in all dropsical persons. It attacks those whose viscera are obstructed, inflamed, ulcerated, or abscessed, and these lesions may be the cause of the fever.

THE TREATMENT OF PECTORAL DROPSY

To a modern reader the third chapter of the Breslau treatise, dealing with therapeutics, is only slightly less bewildering than the second.

At the outset (III. 1) the general purposes of the treatment are set forth. These are: to remove the fluid, to prevent it from forming anew, and to avoid cachexia. These purposes, it is acknowledged, are hard to attain. Riverius said the disease is very serious and hard to cure; Fonseca says it is incurable. Yet some cures are recorded in the literature. Here the tone is sensible and practical.

Venesection offers little hope and may do harm. As to thoracentesis, opinions in the literature vary widely. Riverius had not seen the procedure used and would not recommend it. Salius Diversus was opposed to thoracentesis because it did not solve the main part of the problem, namely to prevent reaccumulation.

With characteristic moderation and good sense the Breslau physicians state that thoracentesis should not be rejected merely because it is an insufficient remedy.

Another objection is of greater weight, i.e., thoracentesis is ineffective against fluid *within* the lung.

Therefore the procedure should not be undertaken "unless it has been established by undoubted signs that there is water fluctuating in the cavity of the chest." The authors quote in extenso the case of Willis, who by means of thoracentesis successfully treated a case of chronic hydrothorax. Vesicants are regarded skeptically. Scarification is useful against edema of the feet and puncture may be used for the swollen scrotum. These all are classed as external remedies.

Among internal remedies (III. 2) first consideration is given to purges, including manna, elaterium, and others; each has its distinguished proponents.

With the diuretics (III. 3) the reader enters the strange world of eighteenth-century pharmacology. Like the modern physician confronted by a case of intractable edema, the Breslau authors wondered which diuretics (and alleged diuretics) should be chosen. They doubted the appropriateness of saline diuretics, since these increase the salinity of the serum and hence supply an increased quantity of the substance which causes relaxation of the kidneys!

They considered it preferable to employ substances which reduce the mucoid character of the fluids, thereby facilitating separation of the thinner part of the serum. Substances that accomplish this are sharp and fatty resins, the root of vincetoxicum, and antiscorbutic plants of all kinds. We are not told why it is believed that these drugs possess such properties. Also commended are the vegetable diuretic water of Willis, an ammoniacal salt, and preparations made from millipedes and bugs.

When fever is complicated by dropsy, the stronger diuretics should be avoided; the reason for this proscription is not stated. Drugs recommended in such cases include perch stones, crab's eyes, and tartar. In the absence of fever, birch beer, radish juice, and berries are useful.

In general, our authors remark, it is dangerous to give diuretics unless laxatives are given first and intercurrently. Diuretics dilate the pores of the kidneys. If purges are not given, a mass of unclean material, containing thick crude sediment, is thrown upon the kidneys and may obstruct them, causing suppression of urine. This statement is typical of the pharmacological sections of the Breslau treatise and seems to be a traditional doctrine gradually elaborated by ratiocination and supported by no truly relevant observational evidence.

Despite this, it must be recognized that the Breslau academicians correctly understood one important part of the therapeutics of hydrothorax, viz. that the physician should attempt to rid the patient of fluid.

From diuretics the discussion turns to diaphoretics (III. 4). These drugs are deemed extremely important in the treatment of dropsy because the body of the dropsical person abounds in serous and vaporous impurities. Further, the blood is viscid.

Diaphoretics thin the blood and fluidify it; likewise they reduce the stickiness of the lymph and they dispel obstructions.

These properties are found in a large variety of drugs, such as theriac waters prepared with spirits, decoctions of guaiac, juniper, and sassafras, and a host of others.

For reasons not stated in the present text, sudorifics were held to be dangerous in the presence of respiratory difficulty. These drugs were deemed especially useful in cases of pruritus and excoriation.

When fever is complicated by dropsy, the authors continue, sudorifics are valuable and should be given repeatedly, e.g., in the form of an electuary of sambucus and crabs' eyes. Diaphoretics are of little direct value for the evacuation of water from the chest but they are useful against fevers, which may cause dropsy.

Pectoral remedies (III. 5) are highly commendable, especially if the lungs are distended by glutinous serum; but, our authors add, it is hard to understand how they could be effective against hydrothorax unless it is assumed that the surface of the lung contains pores through which fluid may pass to the trachea. For pectoral drugs to be effective, cough must be present and there must be mucoid matter in the trachea and bronchi. But the physician should be careful, because expectorants not only cause mucous matter to be ejected from the lung; they may also provoke a flow of mucus *to* the lung and thus endanger the patient.

If evacuation of the peccant matter, i.e., the pleural fluid, has been achieved (III. 6)—and we are not told exactly how this happy result can be recognized— the physician must then turn his attention to correcting, so far as possible, any disorders of the fluids and any visceral inflammations, obstructions, and scirrhi that may be present. For improvement of the fluids a long list of vegetable drugs is suggested, such as absinth, mint, and lesser centaury, as well as certain mineral drugs such as vitriolated tartar and purified niter. These drugs also are useful against obstructions of the viscera. Drugs derived from animals are said to be useless.

The authors now turn to the treatment of special symptoms (III. 7), such as fever and dyspnoea. They quote in extenso a complicated treatment by Pompeius Saccus, based partly on Peruvian bark. Having quoted it, they reject it, since the bark possesses marked astringency, which they have found by experience to be deleterious in fevers of this kind. Indeed, they add, daily experience shows that the bark if given unwisely may even do harm in true intermittent fevers. Here the tone is that of experienced medical practitioners expressing indignation against imprudent therapy.

To these statements they add that the fevers which complicate hydrothorax are due to infarcts, tubercles, scirrhi, and other lesions which block the access of blood. Hence the treatment should consist of deobstruents and resolvents.

How should the physician treat severe and life-threatening respiratory difficulty? The milder medications (III. 8) are useless. The condition contains a convulsive element and this fact may be used in the selection of drugs. Bezoar, antispasmodics, carminatives, and diuretics may be employed.

Tobacco smoke is useful for the treatment of suffocation (!), but its value is difficult to explain. It is generally known that tobacco contains sharp, oily, and salty components; and it opens the pores of ducts, constricts their fibrils, and fluidifies viscid substances. Yet it is not known how this aperient incisive drug is able to stop an impending attack of asthma.

Having discussed in great detail the therapeutics of hydrothorax, the Breslau academicians conclude (III. 9) by confessing that the disease is almost incurable. Often the sick are not only not cured, their symptoms are not even mitigated. In such cases medication should be given sparingly; indeed the physician will not offend against Christianity if he abstains entirely from prescribing.

The eminent Wepfer had tried various drugs on himself. Finding that diuretics annoyed his bladder, he gave up drugs and came to rely on diet alone. Finally, attention should be paid to pure air, peace of mind, open bowels, and sleep. These statements conclude the final chapter of the treatise.

HISTORICAL CONSIDERATIONS

Having reviewed at length the contents of the Breslau monograph, we must now attempt to determine where the essay stands in respect to the development of cardiological knowledge. This is best judged by recapitulation of the concepts of pathogenesis which the authors express or imply.

The text states that fluid enters the pleural cavity from broken vessels and ducts (II. 2) in the chest. It has been demonstrated that there are many lymphatics in this part of the body. Lymph resembles the fluid found in hydrothorax (II. 4); it may enter the chest via obstructed or damaged lymphatic vessels and from broken glands (II. 4). Watery blood sends out serum into the chest (II. 5).

After this recital of anatomical and other causes, which occupies several pages of the printed text, the authors say: "But perhaps it is better to admit frankly that the manner in which serum flows out of the blood vessels and lymphatics cannot be determined accurately … " (II. 5). This avowal does not signify that the authors have given up all attempts to discover the pathogenesis of hydrothorax, since they subjoin an additional series of causes (II. 7–14). They now assert (II. 7) that the cause of the extravasation is to be sought in the fluids, vessels, viscera, or in all together. Inspissation of lymph may rupture the lymphatic vessels or they may become damaged (II. 8) by constriction or compression. The blood emits serum because unfavorable chemical alteration ("dyspepsia") has led to obstructive viscidity (II. 9). Lymph, through delay, may fail to enter and dilute the thick venous blood, and veins may be narrowed by external pressure. Impediments in the circulation (II. 10) may be caused by arterial plaques and polypous concretions. The thoracic duct may break (II. 11). And thoracic congestions, variously caused (II. 13–14), may also lead to hydrothorax.

What are we to make of this system of vague and conflicting etiologies? More precisely, where does this collection of etiologic statements belong in the development of cardiology?

The most conspicuous feature of what we may call the *Breslau pathogenesis* is the virtual absence of any participation by the heart in the production of pleural effusions. While the Harveian doctrine of the circulation is mentioned repeatedly, and while various effects are attributed to sluggishness of the circulation, the concept of defective cardiac function is not mentioned. Indeed the total influence of Harvey's discovery is strangely small.

If the Harveian influence was small, two comparatively recent bodies of research played a more powerful part in the Breslau pathogenesis. One is Lower's experimental production of edema by interruption of venous flow; the direct relevance of this investigation will not be questioned by the modern reader. A second and greater influence was exerted by those anatomists who had studied the lymphatics, especially Nuck and Pecquet. Something about the lymphatic system—perhaps it was the strange appearance of the cisterna chyli or the erratic course of the thoracic duct—seems to have captivated the Breslau academicians and led them to overestimate greatly the role of the lymphatics in the pathogenesis of hydrothorax.

From the mass of doctrines that compose the Breslau pathogenesis we can discern two that seem to preponderate. The first is obstruction, which is mentioned repeatedly as affecting lymphatics, arteries and veins—no differentiation between venous and arterial obstruction being mentioned or even suggested. The obstructive factor is possibly a reflection of the old iatromechanical doctrines. The second factor, inspissation and acridity of the body fluids, is virtually equivalent to chemical alteration and was doubtless inherited from the old humoralism.

With respect to non-cardiogenic hydrothorax, the Breslau physicians correctly point out the tendency of pleural effusions to accompany diseases of the lung. As I have indicated in earlier paragraphs of the present discussion, they mention an almost complete diapason of pulmonary lesions, which they had either observed or read about, such as scirrhous change, callous change, tubercles, hydatids, suppuration, gangrene, and putridity (I. 17), but their statement here takes the form of a summary review and no additional details are supplied, nor is any special speculation presented as to possible pathogenetic relations between hydrothorax and such lesions as scirrhi. It is also interesting that in the recital of the pulmonary lesions that accompany hydrothorax the expected heavy preponderance of tuberculous lesions fails to appear.

Despite the intricacy of their presentation, the Breslau authors are revealed as men of abundant common sense and wide experience. Endowed with considerable knowledge of normal anatomy, almost devoid of applicable physiological knowledge, meagerly instructed in morbid anatomy, and poorly equipped with effective drugs, they were aware of their own limitations and clearly understood that the problem which they confronted could not be overcome by the means then available.

PRACTICAL OBSERVATIONS ON DROPSY OF THE CHEST IN WHICH THE SIGNS, CAUSES, AND METHOD OF TREATMENT OF THIS VERY OBSCURE DISEASE ARE DISCUSSED. ISSUED BY THE LEOPOLDINE ACADEMY OF SCIENTISTS AT BRESLAU

To the Most Sacred, Powerful, and Unconquered Emperor of the Romans, Joseph I, Perpetual August King of Germany, Hungary, Bohemia, Dalmatia, Croatia, Slavonia, Bulgaria, Bosnia, Servia, and Rashka[1]; Supreme Duke of Austria; Duke of Burgundy, Brabant, Styria, Carinthia, Carniola, and of Luxembourg, Württemberg, and Silesia; Count of Tyrol, etc., etc., etc.,

Most August Emperor! When the most glorious Emperor Leopold I the Great was snatched away from earth by a dire fate, amid the unparalleled grief of all Europe, the cities of your subject province of Silesia, and its fields, marketplaces, and crossroads likewise resounded with sad lamentation and wailing. Persons of all ages, sexes, and ranks, animated by feelings of bitter calamity, were in mourning and were steeped in the densest darkness of sorrow. After you, August Emperor, like a rising sun, began to illuminate the people with the rays of your most auspicious regime and began to dispel the darkness with the new light of your majesty, the nations gradually drew their spirits away from the sight of [their] troubles, made an end to lamenting the death of their excellent Prince, and concluded that it was their duty to testify to Leopold their respect for his most faithful spirit—during life he had embraced every divine and human grace—and to prove their devotion. Those who revere studies believed that the death of the Emperor should not be requited with tears, which he had always turned away from them while he lived; but they asserted that his deeds, raised to the skies, should be consecrated to eternity by the voice and letters of the Muses. Some men celebrated his shining piety, which took priority and precedence over all other activities in his life and which he cultivated in his court as well as before the altar. Others commended his unique and rare wisdom and the policy of his profound mind with which the affairs of the Christian world glittered, and his wisdom in arranging present affairs and in predicting the future. Still others with due praises extolled the many magnificent triumphs which he achieved as auspicious victor, who always waged righteous wars, who did not create provinces but defended them, and who did not occupy [the territories] of others but protected his own. Others were found who expressed [the theme] in weighty terms and as elaborately as the subject required. These men transmit the study of literature to posterity. Still others marveled at other virtues in the most glorious Emperor, but all with one voice admitted that no man born, even if he possessed unlimited eloquence, could be found equal to him, [or] could compass the

divine virtues of the great Leopold in mind or even in words.

The voice of our College of the Academy of Scientists at Breslau, which the great Leopold most mercifully protected and honored with special grace, has long been stilled by the bitterness of great grief, and [the College] has been affected and afflicted by limitless suffering, so that it has been unable most humbly to subserve the avowal of its grateful inclination. But recently his death, but recently his fierce illness, was seen by our eyes. Indeed, when we considered that the divine Leopold did not lose glory in death but increased his glory; that he received a terrible fate with mind unperturbed, and on the contrary vanquished and avoided it, and fell like a star that is to rise elsewhere; that he was taken away not from himself and not from us, since Your August Majesty lives and flourishes; [when we considered these things,] we turned our attention away from a study of his death and toward the consideration of that rather rare disease, which physicians call dropsy of the chest, which was fatal both to the Divine Leopold and to Maximilian II, and which few writers have exerted themselves to unravel. In this way our present little work originated, which we have dared to offer to Your Most August Majesty. We do not deny that it is unworthy of Your Majesty, but men who do not have incense make offering to the gods with milk and salt meal, and no one is blamed for worshiping the gods in whatever way he can. Therefore accept this slender gift of paper which we offer with humblest worship and deep spiritual veneration. Look upon it with the milder rays of your clemency and most graciously favor our humble muses with Imperial Grace, after the example of your most glorious father. Your enemies, whose powers you have broken by your heroic deeds, justly fear you, unconquered Emperor, like a lightning bolt of war, and you are the terror of those who disturb the borders of your realms. But your most devoted subjects and those who worship letters you most mercifully gladden and deem worthy of imperial grace. The increase of letters and arts you count as gain; the eagerness for learning you establish with highest authority. For this reason your glory will survive the passing of the centuries and the fame of your most august name shall be transmitted to remote posterity in the field of Mars by the hands of brave soldiers and in the school of Minerva by the minds and writings of the learned. May God long preserve you for Germany, the kingdoms, and the hereditary provinces, and may he keep you safe from all attack by disease. In you, Most Holy Emperor, the world admires the distinctions of your most august ancestors,

---

[1] Now called Novi Pazar, in Yugoslavia.

the courage of Rudolph I, Albert I, and the Fredericks, the glory and happiness of Albert II, Maximilian I, and Charles V, the piety and wisdom of the Ferdinands, the clemency of Maximilian II, the wisdom of Rudolph II, the generosity of Matthew, and the stoutheartedness of the great Leopold, unconquered by difficulties. May all the distinctions which have been scattered among these heroes of the Austrian people shine together in you alone! May God only will that this joy be perpetuated to your subjects! This the most subject servants of your Most August Majesty solemnly desire and pray.

To The Reader, Greetings

The advice concerning the establishment of societies or academies for the advance of [medical] practice which the most distinguished Giorgio Baglivi gave in book II, chapter 4 of his famous book *De Praxi Medica ad Priscam Observandi Rationem Revocanda* (On the Recall of Medical Practice to its Ancient Method of Observation),[2] although it promises rich fruits in clinical medicine, has thus far not been followed by the learned. Nor have we found by discussion that societies of this kind have been established anywhere. Among the principal obstacles which have placed a bar against this most praiseworthy design up to this very time, we would mention—not in the last place—the epidemic which raged in the medical schools a few years ago, a disease whose virtually pathognomonic sign seemed to be a huge aversion and a certain insolent contempt for all the old [knowledge of] medicine, combined with a perpetual itch for innovation. This symptom is quite similar to that which occurs from time to time in pregnant women, who when oppressed by bad coction of the humors, ignore the best and most healthful foods and in place of them feed on coal and ashes. But in fact this illness has not seized all [persons]. Never has our Germany lacked highly outstanding men who with most exact reliability and utmost diligence have explained in their writings whatever has been observed and retained after long experience by the most learned physicians of every age in the most civilized countries concerning the history, habit, progress, resolution, and cure of this or that disease, and the properties, advantages, and disadvantages of medicines and of medical adjuvants, things corroborated by themselves on the strength of wide experience. And these men with no unskilled pencil have depicted the body of medical [knowledge], whose greatest perfection posterity can hope for and promise to itself from learned Baglivian societies of this kind.

Among our numerous occupations we have intended, however inadequately, to imitate the diligence of such men in the present little book on dropsy of the chest. Although we consider our experience hardly sufficient

for the preparation of a more accurate history of this disease, the experience of others, namely of highly learned physicians, has been of use to us. We have repeatedly praised their writings, for we have held in repugnance the custom of those who brazenly avoid citing an author, either so that they should not be deemed to have learned from others or, when they have stealthily gathered the observations of others, they can by this trick avoid the suspicion of plagiarism, or finally that they might use the labors of others for the creation of new hypotheses, with great benefit to their own reputation. That men of this kind very often faithfully copy the studies of others and yet boast that they have derived benefit from no author, we shall elsewhere demonstrate by clear examples. At this place it shall suffice to mention the haughtiness and arrogance of one Barbette.[3] In his preface addressed to the reader he says: "Out of a hundred authors whom I have consulted I have copied out almost nothing, but I have everywhere used my own opinion and judgment." Nevertheless, although this may be true, it is quite clear from book I, chapter I of his book that he begins with a definition of epilepsy that has been taken from Riverius' *Praxis*[4] without any acknowledgment.

We have regularly inserted the testimonies of writers into the text itself [of the present book] and have not thrown them to the bottom or the margins, after the example of several writers who feel that they are observing good sense and neatness in this matter. We have been guided by the example of highly distinguished men, Rolfinck,[5] Conringius,[6] Wepfer,[7] Meibomius,[8] Bohn,[9] Wedel,[10] Schroeckius,[11] Rivinus,[12]

---

[2] Georgius Baglivius, *De Praxi Medica ad Priscam Observandi Rationem Revocanda Libri Duo* (Leyden, 1669), pp. 170–176.

[3] Paul Barbette, *Opera Omnia Medica, Chirurgica et Anatomica* (Geneva, 1704), praefatio.

[4] Barbette, *op. cit.*, p. 5: Epilepsia est convulsio, vel motus partium corporis plerarumque praeternaturalis, cum mentis et sensuum pro tempore plerumque laesione. See also Lazarus Riverius, *Praxis Medica, Editio Ultima* (Leyden, 1660), book 1, chap. 7, p. 75. This sentence is absent from some earlier editions of Riverius.

[5] Werner Rolfinck (1599–1673), anatomist and chemist, author of works on diagnosis and therapeutics.

[6] Hermannus Conringius (1606–1681), practitioner and teacher of medicine in Germany and Scandinavia; early defender of Harvey.

[7] Johann Jakob Wepfer (1620–1695), eminent Swiss physician, noted especially for his contributions to morbid anatomy. His observations on apoplexy (Schaffhausen, 1658) are famous. He is mentioned repeatedly in the present treatise.

[8] Presumably Henricus Meibomius (1638–1700), professor of medicine, history, and rhetoric at Helmstedt; remembered chiefly for his essay on the eyelid (1665).

[9] Johannes Bohn (1640–1718), professor of medicine at Leipzig and dean of the medical faculty; opponent of iatrochemistry; proponent of experimental physiology.

[10] Probably Georg Wolffgang Wedel (1645–1721), author of treatises on drugs and on physiology.

[11] Lucas Schroeckius (1646–1730), author of essays on musk and other drugs, member of the Academy and director of its *Ephemerides*.

[12] Augustus Quirinus Rivinus (1652–1723), professor and dean of the medical faculty at the University of Leipzig.

Major,[13] Schelhammer,[14] Hoffmann,[15] Sachs à Lewenheimb,[16] and others, although there is no reason why we should preserve the same tenor of wording so anxiously or hold on to the same thread of discourse. And although we do not criticize or upbraid the custom of highly learned men who place the words and references of authors in the margins or at the end, we do not disapprove the methods of Johannes Launoius,[17] expressed in the following words:

When they put citations of authors in the margins, a second book is made, facing the first. Then if anyone wants to see the proof of whatever he is reading, he must always turn pages and turn over leaves, and this kind of work occasions annoyance and bother. This method of writing came into fashion a hundred years ago. It is not so esoteric or so mysterious that it could not have been thought of quite easily by the ancients.

We have used the testimonies of others, especially in recounting the phenomena of dropsy of the chest and the treatment, for when we reach the investigation into the causes, everyone including ourselves, as we believe, may be permitted to test out his mental powers and to pursue the causes without reproach, and even to abandon the camp of the ancients. We have humbly added our own experience, obtained in diversified clinical practice.

You see, gentle reader, the bases of this little work, the experience of other physicians and our own. [You see] reason seeking among the phenomena a knowledge of causes, and assuming as its basis the recent discoveries in anatomy. Remember, too, that this book was born amid many activities; rarely has one or other period been finished without interruptions. And so we ask that these writings be judged with the same fairness with which they were written and with which we have judged the works of others, and that your calmness in forgiving be not less than your skill in evaluating. Farewell!

DROPSY OF THE CHEST

CHAPTER I

Showing the History of this Disease

Summary

1. Dropsy of the chest is a disease known to very few.
2. Phenomena which precede the disease, such as precordial oppressions.

---

[13] Johann Daniel Major (1634–1693), professor of anatomy and botany at Kiel.

[14] Guntherus Christophorus Schelhammer (1649–1716), professor at Helmstedt, Jena, and Kiel; wrote extensively on botany, chemistry, and medicine.

[15] Probably the eminent Fridericus Hoffman (1660–1742), professor of medicine at Halle.

[16] Philipp Jacob Sachs von Loewenheim or Lewenheimb (1627–1672), founder of the *Ephemerides Naturae Curiosorum.*

[17] Jean-Piochon de Launay (1649–1701), French surgeon, lithotomist, and monk.

3. Respiration difficult and rapid after the first period of sleep.
4. Pulse often intermittent.
5. Palpitation of the heart. Fainting.
6. Fluctuation of fluid in the chest.
7. Dry cough.
8. Swelling of the scrotum and abdomen.
9. Wasting of the hands.
10. Prodromal fever.
11. Pain in the arms and paralysis. Bloody sputum.
12. Appetite intact.
13. Feces unduly dry. Urine copious and limpid.
14. Death often sudden.
15. Quality of the fluid found in the chest.
16. Its quantity.
17. Condition of the viscera in this disease. Lungs affected unfavorably.
18. Condition of the glands.

1. No physician would deny that water occasionally collects in the lung and in the cavity of the chest, while the other parts of the body and especially the cavities, are either intact, as far as collections of serum, or are affected only secondarily, the region of the chest being affected by dropsy even in the absence of ascites and leukophlegmasia. Dropsy of the chest "is quite difficult to recognize," as Sylvius says in his *Practice,*[18] book I, chap. 50, sect. 25, and "is not described by the majority of physicians and commonly is not detected," according to Riverius[19] in his *Practice of Medicine,* book 7, chap. 5, so that even from the case histories of dropsy of the chest collected by Schenckius,[20] Riverius appropriately concluded that "he had not detected the disease until the cadavers of persons dead of it had been dissected." It is fairly common in Belgium, as Sylvius says in the book already cited, and along the seashores as Köllichen[21] has written in the *Copenhagen Medical and Scientific Reports* (*Acta Medica et Philosophica Hafniensia*). Indeed, nowadays in Germany and other regions fatal cases of this terrible disease occur not rarely. For this reason we shall clearly be doing a worth-while deed if we inquire accurately into its nature, since it has thus far found few writers who have zealously exerted themselves to unravel its characteristics.

2. First of all we must set forth phenomena of this disease that are recognized through the senses, together with circumstances well worth knowing that are suitable for explaining its special character according to the place affected,[22] the times, and the mode of origin. Just as ordinarily happens in ascites, there

---

[18] Franciscus Sylvius, *Praxeos medicae idea nova.* In his *Opera medica* (Amsterdam, 1680), p. 316.

[19] Riverius, *op. cit.* (footnote 4), book 7, chap. 5, p. 458.

[20] Joannes Schenckius a Grafenberg, *Observationum Medicarum Rariorum* (Frankfurt, 1665), book 2, pp. 229 ff.

[21] Caspar Köllichen, "Hydrops Pectoris," *Acta Med. et Philos. Hafniensia* (edited by T. Bartholinus) 2, 118 (1673): pp. 297–298.

[22] While this reference to location reads like an anticipation of Morgagni's *De Sedibus,* it is almost certainly a reflection of the Galenic *De Locis Affectis.*

is a prodromal oppression and discomfort about the precordia. This the patients cannot well express in words and can scarcely describe, and physicians cannot always guess that this precordial discomfort portends a collection of water in the chest.

Half a year ago a French confectionery baker in the court of the Prince died of dropsy of the lungs. A few years before his death, for no manifest reason, he began to have remarkable oppressions, so that he said he did not know what he was doing, like a maniac, and there was danger that he might kill himself. Apart from the paroxysm he was not at all a sad or petulant man; in fact, with his sportive character he was naturally more inclined toward jokes than perhaps was fitting or advantageous. The subsequent events taught us well enough that the cause of his unspeakable anxiety lay hidden not in the hypochondria, as had been thought, but in the chest. In the same way the man from Montpellier, whose thoracic cavity Laurentius[23] found to be full of thick, very red, and very malodorous fluid, had suffered from severe melancholy for three years. See his *Anatomy*, book V, question 13.[24]

3. Further, these patients have severe impediment to respiration, in common with those who have asthma, or ascites, or some other disease of the chest. Hippocrates in *De Morbis*, book 2, n. 59, p. 84, vol. 2[25] says that they breathe ἀθρόον, that is to say *in a crowded manner*; this obviously means difficult, abundant, and frequent respiration, in which the patient seems to be choking. This otherwise does not usually happen in wet asthma, the principal sign of which is correctly stated to be a rather vigorous whistling and noise and a certain sound like a sort of foamy boiling of some kind, with rather laborious respiration, and a sensation of a certain resistance in the lungs. Moreover in this [kind of] asthma a hoarseness or roughness of the voice is ordinarily observed. The situation is different in the dropsy [that we here consider], in which patients are able to express themselves in a loud voice, if matters have not yet come to the end. Indeed the disease we are discussing can easily be distinguished from wet asthma if only we remember that asthmatics of the latter sort can retain a breath of air for a long time without noticeable difficulty and let it out after uttering quite a number of words. People with dropsy [of the chest] cannot do this, since of course it is not easy for them to hold their breath for so long. But

we ourselves rightly doubt whether these [signs] can infallibly distinguish this disease from other similar affections associated with difficulty in breathing.

In our search for another respiratory sign by which this [form of] dropsy can be distinguished from others that are accompanied by difficulty in breathing, nothing else more certain occurs to us than that in dropsy of the chest the respiratory difficulty is so constituted that it oppresses the patient suddenly during the first period of sleep and interrupts his rest, but grants a sort of truce again with the approach of dawn. Before us Carolus Piso made the following splendid statement in his *Selected Observations and Consultations Concerning Diseases Hitherto Overlooked which Arise from Serous Accumulations*,[26] (*Selectae Observationes et Consilia de Praetervisis Hactenus Morbis a Serosa Colluvie Ortis*), sect. 3, chap. 7, p. 296: "It is meet to establish as a pathognomonic sign the difficulty and frequency of respiration which suddenly attacks during the first period of sleep and cheats [the patient] of rest, yet gradually slackens with the advance of the day." On his own account Lazarus Riverius[27] confirms this in book 7, chap. 5, p. 255, already cited above. Apparently we should class with great rarities what is told about a certain young woman in the *Practical Anatomy* of Bonet, book 2, sect. 1, p. 420.[28] Truly from both cavities of the dissected thorax four pounds of stinking water flowed out, yet there had been no orthopnoea or dyspnoea. Heredia[29] in chapter IV of his Dissertation No. 6 on difficult diseases reports that he had seen a man "who was so afraid of his nocturnal attacks of suffocation that he preferred to be worn out by staying constantly awake rather than to compose himself for sleep." Unquestionably our experience has confirmed this in every way. Recently a lady provided us a striking example. Being in danger of suffocation she had called our colleague Dr. Christian Helwich[30] before midnight twice within two weeks. The subsequent swelling of the feet and even of the abdomen, terminated by death, showed clearly enough what disease the difficult and interrupted respiration indicated. It would not be irrelevant in this connection

[23] Andreas Laurentius, *Historia Anatomica Humani Corporis* (Frankfurt, 1600), book 9, quaestio 12, p. 363.

[24] This reference is incorrect. See preceding footnote.

[25] It is evident from the pagination that the Breslau authors were using the version of Hippocrates edited by J. A. van der Linden (Leyden, 1665). For the convenience of the modern reader references to the edition by C. G. Kühn (Leipzig, 1825–1827) will be appended in each instance. The passage in *De Morbis* is at II. 277 ff. in Kühn.

[26] Carolus Piso, *Selectiorum Observationum et Consiliorum De Praetervisis Hactenus Morbis Affectibusque Praeter Naturam ab Aqua seu Serosa Colluvie et Diluvie Ortis* (Leyden, 1714), sect. 3, chap. 7, p. 243. Since I have been unable to discover which edition of Piso the Breslau authors were using, and since it is clear that they did *not* use the original edition (Pont-à-Mousson, 1618), I have regularly supplied footnote references to the convenient edition of Leyden, 1714.

[27] Riverius, *op. cit.* (footnote 4), pp. 459–460.

[28] Theophilus Bonetus, *Sepulchretum sive Anatomia Practica* (Geneva, 1670), book 2, sect. 1, obs. 78, pp. 420–421, appendix: Thoracis hydrops.

[29] Petrus Michaelis de Heredia, *Opera Medica* (Leyden, 1673), 4: disput. 6, chap. 4, p. 71.

[30] Christianus Helwich (1666–1740) physician of Silesian nobility, Stadtarzt at Breslau, author of numerous clinical papers; see also the editor's preface to the present treatise.

to read carefully observations 52, 54 and 55 of Piso,[31] whom we have already praised, and observation 88, century 1[32] of Riverius.

Poterius[33] in Century 1, chapter 2, writes that the exhaled breath of dropsical persons is fetid and even that this disease can be recognized by it. It is uncertain that this man Poterius can safely be trusted, for, according to the illustrious Guy Patin in his first epistle,[34] Poterius' book is "plein de mauvais remedes, de vanteries, de faussettés" (full of bad remedies, boasts, and lies), and Poterius himself was "un grand charlatan et un grand fourbe, qui se meloit de notre metier etc." (a big faker and knave who mixed into our art etc.), as Patin says again. This is certain, that the breath in a cavity is malodorous long before the cavity ruptures.

4. Various kinds of pulse are found in dropsy but it should be noted again and again that [the pulse] is often intermittent. The widow Palearius [sic],[35] who died of dropsy of the lung, "had a large, high, slow, interrupted pulse, which had pauses in one beat and another,"[36] as Ballonius[37] reported in book I of his Epidemics and Ephemerides, p. 17. Rodericus Fonseca says of the dropsical patient discussed in his consultation 54, volume 1,[38] that the pulses were extremely unequal. The pulse of our colleague the eminent Wepfer was generally slow, occasionally unequal, and very often intermittent. For this reason that very experienced man deeply suspected "water or dropsy of the pericardium which impeded cardiac diastole. After his death three pounds of clear water fluctuated in each side of his chest and compressed the lungs, although they floated freely," as his most distinguished son-in-law Dr. Brunner related in the appendix to Year 3, Decuria 3 of the Medico-Physical Ephemerides, pp. 161 and 163.[39] Two years ago, relying on this experience, the eminently praiseworthy Dr. Helwich, in the case of a layman of the Society of Jesus who had shown him his pulse for examination, stated that a collection of serum in the chest was to be feared, because he had found that the pulse was unequal and intermittent. This year the prognosis

was confirmed by the outcome, which was fatal to the patient after he had endured myriads of troubles for about four months.

5. Palpitation of the heart is familiar to many. The sainted Maximilian II offered an outstanding example. Dr. Crato,[40] the Chief Physician, in his oration on the death of Maximilian II spoke as follows, appropriately for our theme: "In our pious deceased emperor, after he had felt palpitation of the heart for more than twenty years, we saw more than two measures of watery fluid left in the cavity of the chest." According to Brunner,[41] Wepfer also felt trembling of his own heart and on this ground the learned Sebizius in his Speculum Medicinae Practicae (Mirror of Practical Medicine), page 892 adds palpitation of the heart to the Hippocratic signs.[42]

With palpitation of the heart lipothymia (fainting) is often combined. The citizen whom we have mentioned above according to Laurentius,[43] for a whole month before his death "was seized twice a day by mild and transient fainting." The Marquis de Finali also, who lived as an exile in the Imperial court and after death had his left thoracic cavity full of dark-red water, had been afflicted not only with various other illnesses but also with dizziness, which is usually combined with fainting; see Schenckius, Observationum Medicarum, book 2, p. 251.[44] And for this reason Willis very appropriately in his Pharmaceutice Rationalis chap. 13, part 2, sect. 1, p. 217 [45] mentions frequent fainting among the diagnostic signs. The three-year-old boy mentioned by Tulpius[46] in his Observations, book 2, chap. 16, page 128, was found after his death to have a chest full of water. He had often had attacks of fainting. In the same place Tulp tells the same story about a thief. Concerning [the case of] a schoolboy see Willis in the place cited above.

6. When there is a large serous collection in the chest, patients complain of its weight pressing the diaphragm down. Therefore it is very hard to draw breath whenever the body must be brought to the

[31] Carolus Piso, op. cit. (footnote 26), sect. 3, chap. 7, obs. 52, p. 237; obs. 54, pp. 239–240; obs. 55, p. 240.

[32] Lazarus Riverius, Opera Medica Universa (Venice, 1713), centuria 1, obs. 88, p. 164.

[33] Petrus Poterius, Insignes Curationes et Singulares Observationes (Cologne, 1624), p. 22.

[34] Guy Patin, Lettres Choisies (Paris, 1685), p. 3.

[35] Ballonius, vide infra, gives the name as Platearius.

[36] Possibly in one beat after another. The text connotes some kind of pulsus alternans.

[37] Gulielmus Ballonius, Epidemiorum et Ephemeridum Libri Duo (Paris, 1640), book 1, p. 17.

[38] Rodericus à Fonseca, Consultationes Medicae (Venice, 1619–1622), consult. 54, 1: p. 197.

[39] Johannes Conradus Brunner, "Memoria Wepferiana." Appendix ad Annum Tertium Decuriae III Ephemeridum Medico-Physicarum Academiae Caesareo-Leopoldinae Naturae Curiosorum (Nuremberg, 1696), pp. 153–168) (see pp. 161, 163).

[40] Johann Crato von Krafftheim, (1519–1585). According to Jonas Graetzer, Lebensbilder hervorragender schlesischer Aerzte (Breslau, Schottlaender, 1889), pp. 15, 19, Crato wrote an Epistola ad Sambucum de Morte Imperatoris Maximiliani II (Frankfurt, 1577),

[41] Brunner, op. cit. (footnote 39), p. 161: Sub sterno tempore paroxysmi constrictionem quasi spasmodicam, cordisque tremorem . . . sensit. (At the time of the paroxysm he felt a sort of spasmodic constriction beneath the sternum and a trembling of the heart.)

[42] Kühn II. 277 ff.

[43] Laurentius, op. cit. (footnote 23), book 9, quaestio 12, p. 363.

[44] Joannes Schenckius a Grafenberg, Observationum Medicarum Rariorum (Frankfurt, 1665), p. 231. The page number given in the Breslau text is incorrect.

[45] Thomas Willis, Pharmaceutice Rationalis, Pars Secunda (London, 1675), sect. 1, chap. 13, p. 233.

[46] Nicholas Tulpius, Observationes Medicae, Editio Nova (Amsterdam, 1652), book 2, chap. 16, pp. 128–129.

erect position or moved. There is also pain in the back—patients point out its location—at the region where the diaphragm is attached to the loins. Fluctuation of water when the body is bent is even perceived by touch. Hippocrates in the *De Morbis* already cited, book 2, page 85, says: "If the ear is put to the sides for a long time you may hear that there is bubbling inside, as if it were vinegar."[47] And this happens when water sticks in the lungs and indeed when it floods the cavity of the chest, as "a sound is perceived which is made by watery fluid enclosed in a half filled leatherbottle," according to Zacutus Lusitanus[48] in book 1, observation III of his *Praxis Admiranda.* However in order for dropsy of the chest to be distinguished more accurately from empyema, it must be skillfully considered whether the patient has previously suffered the illnesses which this condition usually follows, such as whooping cough, angina, pleuritis, peripneumonia, cavitary ulceration of the lungs, penetrating wounds of the chest, concussion, and the like. In fact, one must not even stop here but those conditions must also be weighed which usually follow empyema. For instance it should be discovered whether much sweat is spread over the whole body, whether the patient sometimes has a chill afterward, whether he has pain about the chest, whether the nostrils become narrowed during respiration and the breath whistles as it is drawn through them, whether a rosy color suffuses the face, and whether the palms and soles are hot. If these and other signs of empyema are absent, dropsy can more certainly be deduced from the weight and fluctuation of the material in the chest. Moreover, as Hippocrates says in the treatise already cited,[49] "if you pour anything [on the chest] or use a poultice or fumigation, pus does not follow and from this you will know that water is there, and not pus."

7. With the presence of this material in the chest there is cough, which occurs without expectoration, i.e., dry and such that nothing is expectorated even if the cough is frequent and strong. External swelling we do not remember seeing except in a member of a religious order whom we have already mentioned. He repeatedly showed us his swollen left side. Caspar Bauhinus, quoted by Schenck[50] (*loco citato*, p. 252) tells of a cobbler who suffered from dropsy of the chest; he had "on his back at the left side, a fleshy swelling which did not differ from the skin in color. After emollients applied for a long time had ceased to be effective, a barber opened it with a knife, and water dripped out." In the forty-year old man described by Fonseca[51] (*loco citato*, p. 374) "the hypochondria were swollen on both sides."

8. It happens quite often that with the passing of time the water goes down into the scrotum and makes the genital regions swell. A distinguished gentleman is still alive in whom all signs prove that he is suffering from dropsy of the chest. His scrotum, distended by an immense hydrocoele, had become burdensome to him. On account of the annoyance he recently entrusted himself to a surgeon for puncture. On repeated occasions nearly four pounds of water were let out, not counting that which burst forth vigorously and soaked the dressings, and this amounted to a great deal more. It is very much worth noting that in this kind of dropsy the scrotum becomes swollen before the abdomen or the feet. We have found not once but repeatedly that when the scrotum was already swollen the feet finally were seized with edematous swelling, whence the marvellous harmony between the genital regions and the thorax is again apparent, as observed by Hippocrates[52] and also by us elsewhere in people who had coughs. Just as in ascites, the signs of this swelling in the feet reveal themselves about the malleoli while it gradually increases and climbs up to the knees and even as far as the thighs. In fact, not even the abdomen remains immune to this flood. Day by day it becomes more greatly distended by the watery fluid and indeed even the face swells. Hippocrates[53] (*loco citato*, p. 85) says that "some people swell in the belly, scrotum, and face." For a certain period of time the annoyances are partly alleviated, while waters are pouring out into the abdomen and are making it swell. The patients meanwhile congratulate themselves on the improvement in their health. But in truth the joy is brief, because when the abdomen is filled the symptoms are aggravated.

Fonseca in the book already cited states that his patient's lower lids were swollen. We have seen swelling of the hand and even of the arm in one patient or another. As that most learned gentleman Petrus Salius Diversus[54] writes in chapter 5 of his book on special diseases, page 246, "afterward even the face and scrotum and abdomen become obviously swollen, the watery fluid which is excessively abundant having poured out not only into the chest but into all these regions," although in that passage the discussion is mainly about dropsy.

9. But indeed it not rarely happens that the upper regions, even the hands, waste away while the lower become swollen. On page 163 of his memoir Brunner[55]

[47] Kühn II. 277.

[48] Abraham Zacutus Lusitanus, *De Praxi Medica Admiranda,* book 1, obs. 111. In his *Praxis Historiarum,* (Leyden, 1644), second pagination, p. 26.

[49] *De Morbis.* Kühn II. 277.

[50] Joannes Schenckius a Grafenberg, *Observationum Medicarum Rariorum* (Frankfurt, 1665), book 2, pp. 231–232.

[51] Fonseca, *op. cit.* (footnote 38) 1: p. 197.

[52] Hippocrates: *Epidemics II.* Kühn III. 431.

[53] Kühn II. 277.

[54] Petrus Salius Diversus, *De Febre Pestilenti Tractatus, et Curationes Quorundam Particularium Morborum* (Hardwick, 1656), pp. 245–246.

[55] Brunner, *op. cit.* (footnote 39), p. 162.

noted that this had happened to his father-in-law Dr. Wepfer. Here it is appropriate to look back to Hippocrates and his frequently quoted passage on page 84: "the nails become curved and contracted,"[56] doubtless because at that very place the fleshy parts which lie under the nails waste away, hence it must happen that the nails become extended to greater length and easily become contracted. The same thing happens in consumptives.[57] Franciscus du Port, taught by experience, writes in his second book on the signs of diseases,[58] that the nails in confirmed phthisic and hectic cases become curved and long, like claws of a bird.[59] Compare with the authors of the *Bibliotheca Anatomica*, volume 1, in the notes on Malpighi's treatise *De Cornuum Vegetatione*.[60]

10. In addition the author of the book *De Morbis*, which goes under the name of Hippocrates, intimates that pectoral dropsy can be recognized by fever; indeed he puts fever in first place among the signs. He says, "if there is dropsy in the chest the patient has fever and cough." And we are convinced by experience that this is sometimes the case. In the dropsical case mentioned by Fonseca,[61] "there was a certain lingering fever." Piso[62] likewise, observation 54, page 292, detected in an ecclesiastic "conspicuous swelling in either hypochondrium, but especially in the right, together with intense fever." According to Coiter, [John] Peregrinus, seized with this [i.e., pectoral] dropsy, fell into a hectic marasmus.[63] The Jesuit brother already mentioned also had fever, hence his regular physician suspected that nothing was at the bottom of it but a febrile cattarrh. The primipara discussed by Nicolaus Chesneau of Marseilles in book 5, case 9,[64] about whose sickness the physicians had disagreed while she was still alive, "not only had fever on the day before the delivery. On the very day of the delivery a higher fever appeared; together with a chill and pain in the side it lasted until her death." The forty-five-year-old surgeon who was excessively given to the drinking of wine and who used to feel a sort of overflowing when

he turned from one side to another, had more fever than other symptoms; see Pompeius Saccus[65] in *Medicina Theorico-Practica*, consultation 29, page 114 and consultation 27, where he treats expressly of fever accompanying dropsy of the lungs.

Others suffering from this [kind of] dropsy are free from fever, as we have noticed time and again. The boy described by Piso[66] in his observation 51 had "inspiratory difficulty which gradually increased, equally without fever and without orthopneic cough." Petrus Salius Diversus, *loco citato* p. 246,[67] says "fever is added by the author of the book *De Morbis*[68] but those I treated had no fever." But what he adds is worthless and goes against experience: "by reason of the material, which is [humorally] cold and does not putrefy, fever should not be present." Fernel in book 5, chapter 11 of his *Pathologia*[69] teaches that "this disease presents signs and symptoms of suppuration, except that fever does not occur," or as Jacotius[70] warns, "not so acutely," which, as we have stated, is contrary to experience.

11. As a culmination of trouble, pain in the arms and paralysis[71] are sometimes added, and this noteworthy loosening [of fibers] Carolus Piso[72] has considered, page 293, in the case of the Canon already praised, and, through Piso, Riverius[73] page 255. But to all these signs we judge that one more should be added, namely that [the patients] tolerate heat with difficulty and very easily become cold. This very day an example came before our eyes in [the case of] the distinguished gentleman whom we have already mentioned in the same way; in the very same season when it is summer and we are roasting and everyone is uncomfortable, he complains of cold even in bed. And as for Wepfer, Brunner[74] witnessed that "he easily became cold, especially in his extremities."

Among the rarest phenomena of this disease is bloody sputum, which Saccus, who has been praised in a preceding paragraph, noticed in that dropsical surgeon of his. Perhaps it happens more often that dropsy follows the expectoration of blood; concern-

---

[56] The text is given both in Greek and in Latin translation. Kühn II. 277.

[57] Lat. *tabidi*, persons wasted by disease, usually but not necessarily what we now call tuberculosis.

[58] François Duport, *De Signis Morborum Libri Quattuor* (Paris, 1584), book 2, chap. 23, p. 43 and p. 44, n. 19.

[59] *Veluti alitis ungues.* Regrettably this impressive simile is not used nowadays in teaching.

[60] Daniel Leclerc and Jean Jacques Manget, *Bibliotheca Anatomica* (Geneva, 1685) 1; pp. 38–39.

[61] Fonseca, *op cit.* (footnote 38), p. 197.

[62] Piso, *op. cit.* (footnote 26), sect. 3, chap. 7, obs. 54, pp. 239–240.

[63] Volcher Coiter, *Externarum et Internarum Principalium Humani Corporis Partium Tabulae* (Nuremberg, 1572). Reprinted in Opuscula Selecta Neerlandicorum de Arte Medica **18** (1955); see pp. 134–135).

[64] Nicolaus Chesneau, *Observationum Medicarum Libri Quinque* (Paris, 1672), book 5, obs. 9, pp. 500–508.

[65] Pompeius Saccus, *Medicina Theorico-Practica* (Parma, 1687), pp. 114 and 107–109.

[66] Piso, *op. cit.* (footnote 26), sect. 3, chap. 6, p. 235.

[67] Diversus, *op. cit.* (footnote 54), p. 246.

[68] Kühn II. 277.

[69] Joannes Fernelius, *Pathologia*, book 5, chap. 11, p. 158. In his *Medicina* (Paris, 1554).

[70] Desiderius Jacotius Vandoperamus, author of treatises on various Hippocratic writings, including the *Coaca Praesagia* (Leyden, 1576) and *De Morborum Internorum Curatione* (Paris 1567).

[71] Lat. *paralysis* sometimes signifies numbness and not motor disability.

[72] Piso, *op. cit.* (footnote 26), sect. 3. chap. 6, obs. 51, p. 235.

[73] Lazarus Riverius, *Praxis Medica* (Leyden, 1660), book 7, chap. 5, p. 460.

[74] Brunner, *op. cit.* (footnote 39), p. 161.

ing this occurrence the same Saccus composed a consultation, Consilium 28.[75]

12. As to the appetite for food, it is intact not only in the beginning but also occasionally during the progress and increase of the disease, and no huge thirst is present. But experience thus far has taught that food ingested in rather large quantity arouses an asthmatic paroxysm. This was experienced by Wepfer, whom we have mentioned rather often; and that old man of illustrious position, in this respect very similar to Wepfer, experienced it repeatedly, but "[this gentleman] could take food only while he was erect, and very little food—although he had appetite— through fear of an asthmatic paroxysm which was excited even by eating." The religious woman mentioned by Johannes Chiffletius,[76] observation 16, p. 24, had dined well before her death.

13. In many [patients] the excrements are discharged from the body duly and in the proper way. You may find, in those who move their bowels, in some patients the stool is drier than it should be, the flow of urine is copious and natural, and morning sweats follow as desired. From repeated experience we know that thin clear urine poured forth in large quantities indicates that an asthmatic paroxysm is imminent. The confectionary baker whom we have mentioned in a previous section sometimes would pass very large amounts of pale urine and sometimes very scanty and well colored urine, so that the distinguished Sorbait,[77] Med. Pract. tract. 1, chap. 58, is not at all wrong when he teaches that "urines of this kind, if they are voided often, portend dropsy." When the disease is getting worse the urine is scantier and mostly darker and thicker. In those who have consulted us and were near death, we have noted urine reddish to black, with a sediment which resembled bran or brickdust.

14. This disease is chronic and often punishes the patients miserably for many years. When they have reached the point where no hope remains, they do not immediately die. With groans and tears they draw breath for a long time, as long as nature, and art, the rival of nature, contrive with some success the depletion of water through pathways suited to the movement of serum, namely the stool, the urinary passages and the pores of the body. But when these evacuations fail, the thread of life is not [always] broken in the same way. Some die unexpectedly as if suffocated. Thus, a few weeks ago a certain man

who for many years had spent his nights getting up again and again, set out for a wedding and suddenly suffocated. The sixty-year old patient of Blanckard,[78] Practical Rational Anatomy, book 1, case 98, "suddenly fell down in unexpected death as if he had been hit by lightning." We have found that many die as if finished off by marasmus. Another patient of Blanckard's,[79] century 2, observation 48, died from loss of strength after he had suffered for a long time from asphyxia. We remember having seen someone who on the day of that funeral, when the world was abandoned,[80] had repeated convulsions but seemed perfectly well to the bystanders. Nevertheless he suddenly lost his voice and died like an apoplectic. Those persons depart from this life with greater trouble who are afflicted with aversion to food and with vomiting for some days before or who occasionally give up a little clear water by mouth. This is proof that the flood of serum has metastasized to the stomach, through unknown pathways.

15. These things are observed in living people partly from the reports of patients and partly from direct observation. To these must be added the things which are revealed in the dead by means of the anatomist's knife. And indeed, if you look at the fluid, that which is found after death in the dissected thorax is not always the same. At times the water is found to be entirely liquid, and resembles pure water in color. A memorable instance is found in Piso's book[81] at the place already mentioned, section 3, chapter 7 in that Canon whose whole chest was found "full of pure water in a stupendous amount." Compare also Michinus[82] in observation 7 of his appendix to the commentary of Fallopius on Galen's book on bones.[83]

In the chest of a certain Belgian "the tunic of the lungs closely adherent on either side to the pleura and beneath to the diaphragm had formed a number of huge hydatids full of water, which like a fountain, had flooded the right side of the thorax with a large amount of water and had caused dropsy of the chest," according to [Thomas] Bartholinus[84] in century 2, history 66, page 291 of his Historiarum Anatomicarum. Sometimes moreover the water is mucilaginous and when fire is applied it clots into gelatin. Of this kind was the water which was drained away from a living young man by paracentesis performed in the presence of Lower and Willis. To use the words of

---

[75] Pompeius Saccus. See above (footnote 65), consilium 28, p. 110–113.

[76] Johannes Chiffletius. The British Museum General Catalogue of Printed Books (London, 1966) 38: col. 312 lists the following, to which I have not had personal access: Chifflet, Jean: Ioannis Chiffleti . . . Singulares tam ex curationibus, quam cadauerum sectionibus obseruationes (Paris, I. Richer, 1612).

[77] Paul Sorbait, Tractatus Primus Physiologo-Practicus, chap. 58, p. 375. In his Universa Medicina, tam Theorica quam Practica (Nuremberg, 1672).

[78] Stephen Blancardus, Anatomia Practica Rationalis (Amsterdam, 1688), book 1, obs. 98, pp. 189–190.

[79] Blanckard, pp. 265–266.

[80] Perhaps the day of the Emperor's funeral.

[81] Piso, op. cit. (footnote 26), sect. 3, chap. 7, pp. 239–240.

[82] This name is misspelled Minchin[us] in the Breslau original.

[83] Franciscus Michinus, Expositio in Librum Galeni de Ossibus (Venice, 1570), pp. 75–76.

[84] Thomas Bartholinus, Historiarum Anatomicarum Rariorum Centuria I et II (Amsterdam, 1654), centuria 2, historia 66, p. 263.

the latter, "a thick fluid came out, whitish as chyle and almost milky."[85]

Bloody serum has been found in many other patients. Rondeletius[86] especially saw it in the chest of a certain merchant; [see] book 2 of his Method[us] Curand[orum], chapter 24, page 387. Occasionally it verges somewhat on yellow, like natural urine or lye. "In a certain seven-year old girl who suffered from measles the cavity of the chest was full of citrinous fluid," according to Bonetus[87] in book 2, page 427 of the book previously cited. The water which filled the left cavity of the chest of Marquis de Finali resembled lye in quality and color as Schenck says in quoting a case of Aicholtz. [Hieronymus] Faber, a Bavarian physician, saw greenish fluid, as reported by Schenck[88] on page 253. There are even some men who say they have seen black fluid, and among them is Coiter. Stephanus Blanckard[89] saw greenish-yellow fluid; [see his] Anatomia Practica Rationalis, century 1, case 98. According to Hercules de Saxonia,[90] art. 1, chap. 26, several pounds of foamy water which showed signs of viscidity were found in the cavity of the thorax and in the lungs of a certain man of the Marcellus family.

There is no doubt of the saltiness and bitterness of the water. In a hospital the distinguished Sylvius dissected a girl about twenty years old in whose right thoracic cavity especially there was copious water, "and from the acrimony of this water the pleura and the entire inner surface of the diaphragm were ulcerated and eroded, so that they even yielded pus," Dr. Brechtfeld tells from his own observation in our Ephemerides.[91] This acrimony was confirmed by the tongues of bystanders and tasters when Borrichius dissected a man who had died of triple dropsy; Acta Hafniensia, vol. 1, p. 174.[92]

The water which floods the chest is not only very bitter but at times it is also fetid. In the dissected body of a Parisian notary "there were found ten Paris pounds[93] of serous fluid, putrid and malodorous, moving about in the whole chest." Not less fetid was the abundant fluid [in the case] of the girl whom we have already mentioned. That the fluid sometimes is mixed with purulent material is stated in all anatomical histories, especially those of Caspar

Bauhinus; and Salmuth,[94] centuria 1, obs. 13, noticed a very bad smell when he was opening the body of a young man whose thorax poured forth a great abundance of fluid. Lungs containing purulent cavities and distended with caseous substance are mentioned by Harder in the scholia of his observations on practical anatomy, observation 51.[95]

16. The quantity of this serous fluid is variable. Sometimes the water effused into the thorax weighs several pounds, as may become evident from what has been said above. In the case of De Clerck two pounds were found on the right side according to Otto Heurnius, observation 6.[96] Fourteen pounds were found in the right chest of a cobbler, according to testimony of Oethaeus in Schenckius.[97] Indeed sometimes it is so abundant that it can fill several brass vessels. As Bauhinus says, from the thorax of a cobbler "purulent fluid [enough to fill] three brass pots flowed out of his right chest; on this side the whole lung had turned into pus while the left lung remained intact." Sometimes both cavities of the chest are filled and by the abundance of water in one woman "the diaphragm, in the region where the esophagus passes, had been pushed like a sac against the left kidney" according to Harderus[98] on page 217 of the Apiarium and, what will astound you, at times "such a quantity of fluid is collected within the cavern of the chest that it cannot be restrained, but a huge quantity of this serum enters the abdominal space" which before our time Jacotius noted in his comments on Hippocrates, and before Jacotius Hippocrates himself noted in book II of Diseases (De Morbis).[99] In fact the fluid even fills the lungs themselves and occupies the bronchi, or the whole lung "is weighed down and imbued" with serum of this kind, as was noted by the famous Lucas Tozzi.[100] "In the cadaver [of a person] who had died of this kind of sickness the lung was so distended and swollen with glutinous serum that it occupied all the space in the chest" as Tozzi[101] himself reports in Medicina Practica p. 309 et seq. So that there should be no lack of those who with Hippocrates advise that a distinction be drawn between dropsy of the lung and dropsy of the chest, Melchior Sebizius[102] in the Speculum Medicinae Practicae, part 3, section 3,

---

[85] Thomas Willis, Pharmaceutice Rationalis. Pars Secunda (London, 1675), sect. 1, chap. 13, pp. 230-231.

[86] Gulielmus Rondeletius, Methodus Curandorum Omnium Morborum (Frankfurt, 1592), book 2, chap. 24, p. 287.

[87] Bonetus, op. cit. (footnote 28), book 2, sect. 1, 1: p. 427.

[88] Joannes Schenckius a Grafenberg, Observationum Medicarum Rariorum (Frankfurt, 1665), book 2, p. 232.

[89] Blanckard, op. cit. (footnote 78), centuria I, obs. 98, p. 189.

[90] Hercules Saxonia, Pantheum Medicinae Selectum (Frankfurt, 1603), book 2, chap. 8, p. 179.

[91] I have been unable to find Brechtfeld's report.

[92] Olaus Borrichius, Anatome Centurionis Triplici Hydrope Enecti. In Thomae Bartholini Acta Medica et Philos. Hafniensia Ann. 1671 et 1672 (Copenhagen, Haubold, 1673) 1: pp. 173-174.

[93] The old French livre is equivalent to 489.5 gm.

[94] Philippus Salmuth, Observationum Medicarum Centuriae Tres (Brunswick, 1648), centuria 1, obs. 13, p. 10. Salmuth mentions no odor in his report.

[95] J. Harderus, Apiarium (Basle, 1687), pp. 216 ff. The Breslau text is slightly obscure at this point.

[96] Otto Heurnius, Historiae et Observationes Quaedam Rariores ex Praxi et Diario. Historia 6, p. 12. Appended to J. Fernelius, Universa Medicina (Utrecht, 1656).

[97] Schenckius, op. cit. (footnote 20), book 2, pp. 231-232.

[98] Harderus, 1687, p. 217.

[99] Kühn II. 277.

[100] Lucas Tozzi [1638-1717], iatrochemist, Hippocratic commentator, professor of medicine at Naples.

[101] Lucas Tozzi, Medicina Praktike (Bologna, 1697), p. 237.

[102] Melchior Sebizius [junior], Manualis, sive Speculi Medicinae Practici (Argentorati, 1661), part 3, sect. 3, chap. 13, 1: p. 892.

chap. 13, mentions himself among those [who hold this opinion].

Dropsy of the pericardium is often associated with this flood in the lungs and thorax. You may like to hear what Olaus Borrichius says about a centurion in the passage already cited.[103] "In the chest," says he, "a new source of catastrophe disclosed itself, for the lungs were small, dry, flaccid, and, except for their extreme margins, half putrid; and they floated about in very abundant foul fluid. Moreover, what was almost a wonder, the pericardium was so broadened and distended as to enclose three pounds and more of sharp turbid liquid in its cavity." So you learn from this that confidence should not so rashly be withdrawn from Cornelius Stalpart van der Wiel,[104] when he reports in cent. 1, obs. 36, p. 144 *et seq.* shaking of water in the pericardium "in a poor little cachectic girl of seventeen years, whose pulsating heart could even be heard externally" since at other times the pericardium naturally contains no more than about two or three spoonfuls, according to several [authors]. And although this fluid is not secreted and accumulated except in extreme conditions and at the last moment of life, finally on account of rather violent movements of the heart and obstructed circulation through the lungs, in those who die stabbed and beheaded or without noteworthy disturbance of the circulation, certainly no fluid is found, as is asserted and shown, together with other facts, by the most distinguished Bohnius[105] in *De Renunciatione Vulnerum*, pp. 307-309.

17. After considering the fluid, we must very briefly discuss in what way the viscera are disposed in this [kind of] dropsy. In the first place the lungs obtrude themselves [on our attention] because they are commonly affected in an unfavorable way. Wepfer's lungs[106] were "compressed but floating freely in water and were quite inflated, so that he seemed to have died during inspiration rather than in expiration." Many have found the lungs hard and dry. Michinus[107] noticed that "they were scirrhous or callous." Carolus Piso,[108] section 3 of chapter 8, found them "parched and full of purulent gore, and one of the lungs was quite completely dried out." Hippocrates found tubercles and hydatids, as did many later writers. Observers report the lungs to have been "partly consumed and corrupted." Harderus[109] in his case 51, page 215, writes the follow-

ing about a certain eighteen-year-old woman: "the right lung was everywhere very tightly adherent and united to the ribs. The left was a little less completely affected, and the entire left [pleural] cavity was seen to be full of a greenish fluid resembling water spoiled by long stagnation, to the measure of about a pound. In the lowest part of this fluid there were thick and whitish deposits, real pus. What remained of the left lung was a thin stump sprinkled variously with foul ulcers." In the man mentioned by Blanckard[110] on page 265 of the treatise already cited, the left lung was entirely putrid; and in the woman described by Harderus[111] "the lungs were clearly consumed by rot." Edmundus de Meara[112] in his *Historiae Medicae Rariores*, p. 136, even saw gangrenous lungs. The neighboring parts of the lungs also are not immune from destruction. For it can be read here and there that the pleura "was thick and callous" and that the same faults had affected the mediastinum, the diaphragm, and other structures.

In like manner the pericardium has its own fates. In the cadaver of De Clerck its substance, as Heurnius[113] states, "was fleshy rather than membranous and six times thicker than natural, and firmly united to the heart so that it could not be separated from it by the fingers without tearing." Highly noteworthy is the fact that the most distinguished Professor Zellerus[114] of Tübingen found in a garrison soldier who had died of dropsy in the chest that the entire pericardium was full "of lentil-sized granules" with which the entire internal layer was roughened, "although it contained eleven ounces of water." The destruction creeps even as far as the very source of life, the heart, whose vessels occasionally are full of black blood. Wepfer's heart was "speckled and reddish near the conus intertriginis; the left chamber (ventricle) of the heart contained a few little masses and pure fluid blood. In the base of the heart near the pulmonary artery a bony substance came against the knife. The aorta behind the semilunar valves with its bony roughness caught the entering fingers." These [are the statements of] Brunner,[115] whose remaining remarks about the ossification of the aorta are worthy of being read and pondered in practice.

Sometimes the viscera in the abdomen are found to be obviously normal, as in the cadaver of Clerck,[116]

[103] Borrichius, *op. cit.* (footnote 92), p. 174.

[104] Cornelius Stalpart van der Wiel, *Observationum Rariorum Medic. Anatomic. Chirurgicarum* (Leyden, 1687), centuria 1, obs. 36, pp. 144–145. Quassatio aquae in pericardio, etiam foris auribus percepta.

[105] Johannes Bohnius, *De Renunciatione Vulnerum, seu Vulnerum Lethalium Examen* (Leipzig, 1689), pp. 307–309.

[106] Brunner, *op. cit.* (footnote 39), p. 163.

[107] This name is misspelled *Minchinus* in the Breslau text. See above, footnotes 82 and 83.

[108] Piso, *op. cit.* (footnote 26), sect. 3, chap. 8, p. 249.

[109] J. Harderus, *op. cit.* (footnote 95), obs. 51, p. 215.

[110] Blanckard, *op. cit.* (footnote 78), centuria 2, obs. 48, pp. 265–266: Thorace aperto, ingens aquae foetentis copia effluxit, pulmo sinister putridus. When the chest was opened, a large amount of fetid water flowed out; the left lung was putrid.

[111] Harderus, *op. cit.* (footnote 95), p. 217.

[112] Edmundus de Meara, *Examen Diatribae Thomae Willisii . . . Cui Accesserunt Historiae Aliquot Medicae Rariores* (Amsterdam, 1667), p. 134.

[113] Heurnius, *op. cit.* (footnote 96).

[114] Johann Gottfried Zeller [1656–1734]. Source not identified.

[115] Brunner, *op. cit.* (footnote 39), p. 163.

[116] Heurnius, *op. cit.* (footnote 96).

excepting the omentum alone, "which was withered and black, and the gall bladder, in which there were three stones." The Canon, whom we have repeatedly mentioned after Piso,[117] "had a swollen, hard, parched liver, like a fragment of pumice, and pitted." When Borrichius[118] opened the cadaver of a centurion "the spleen was found to be four times larger than the normal, harder than natural, and swollen here and there with a kind of black sediment." It is known also from the experience of many that ulcerated and putrid kidneys have been found in these dropsical persons. The stomach and intestines also share the evil. And not to speak of the various affections of the alimentary canal, it is very likely that water sometimes waves about in this entire canal. Costerus[119] observed this in a dropsical patient.

18. The rarity of the case reports of Otto Heurnius,[120] which are appended to the works of Fernel, persuades us to excerpt here several items from his history 10, page 8, which splendidly reveal how the glands all over the body behave in dropsical persons. The learned gentleman dissected a fourteen-year-old girl from Leyden whose right chest and abdomen were full of yellowish water. The pericardium likewise was swollen with so much of this fluid, but a little clearer, that the fluid burst forth violently from the incision. The mesentery, omentum, and pancreas abounded with innumerable rather large glands. These were found in large numbers even in the peritoneum, diaphragm, mediastinum, and uterine ligament; some were as big as chestnuts, others as big as filberts, and others as big as peas. At the upper end of the stomach Heurnius noticed two of the size and shape of acorns. There was a large one over the trunk of the portal vein. The liver, spleen, and lung, in addition to rather large glands which were here and there, were completely strewn inside and out, as if by hail. Many that were scarcely larger than a grain of millet or coriander could be seen in the tunics of the intestines, and there was a small one of the same kind in each kidney. In the right side of the dura he found one as big as a pea, which had adhered to the inner table of the cranium and had produced in it the traces of caries. The material contained in them was serous and resembled the dugs of cows or sheep. These and other things are reported by Heurnius in the place [previously] cited.

---

[117] Piso, *op. cit.* (footnote 26), sect. 3, chap. 8, obs. 54, pp. 239–240.

[118] Borrichius, *op. cit.* (footnote 92), pp. 173–174.

[119] Apparently a reference to Johannes Costerus [1613–1676], *Affectuum Totius Corporis Humani* (Frankfurt, 1664).

[120] Heurnius, *op. cit.* (footnote 96), historia 10, p. 14. The Breslau authors have erred as to the page.

CHAPTER II

The Causes of Dropsy of the Chest

Summary.

1. Sources of the disease. Ebullition of blood.
2. Vessels in the chest broken apart.
3. [The cause is] not the nerve fluid—
4. but fluid raining down from the lymphatic vessels into the thorax.
5. Serum exuding from vessels into the cavity of the chest.
6. Chyliferous ducts within the chest broken apart.
7. Where the cause of the extravasation of lymph is to be looked for.
8. Flaws in the lymphatic vessels of other organs.
9. Reasons as to the place from which the blood sends forth serum from its vessels into the cavity of the chest.
10. Ossification of vessels.
11. Chyle poured out of the thoracic duct.
12. Dropsy of the pericardium.
13. More special diseases of the viscera.
14. Which temperaments are suitable for dropsy of the chest.
15. Annoyance and troublesome pain in the precordia.
16. Unequal and occasionally intermittent pulse; its origin.
17. Origins of lipothymia.
18. Cough, whence?
19. Fever a companion of dropsical persons.
20. Coldness of external parts in dropsical people.

1. Order requires that we investigate the origin and generation of this disease. And the hinge of the matter turns on this, that we reveal those sources whence that serous fluid comes which collects in the thorax and after collecting causes dropsy of the chest and commonly wells up. There has been no lack of learned physicians—and among them is Willis[121]—who, when they thought about the subject carefully, considered it not improbable that blood boils quite vigorously in the precordia and that from the boiling blood abundant vapors are produced. If their exhalation is impeded and they are shut up in an enclosure, just as happens in an alembic, these vapors condense into water. The latter, accumulating gradually, produces this [kind of] dropsy. But with all respect to such a great man, this cause is too common and general; and if it is assumed, dropsy is not necessarily assumed. Certainly if dropsy were produced in this way it would be wonderful how any of the animals which breathe could escape this disease for any length of time, since in these animals the boiling of the blood in the precordia is so much more violent and hence the production of vapor is greater.[122]

2. Further, at these times the liquid is sufficient, and nothing comes down from the head through the trachea into the cavity of the chest, although at other

---

[121] Thomas Willis, *Pharmaceutice Rationalis, Pars Secunda* (London, 1675), sect. 1, chap. 13, p. 228.

[122] An excellent example of the type of disputation common in that era. Note also the reference to comparative anatomy.

times we are aware of the synthimony (agreement) described by Duretus between the head and the lungs, "by which they exchange services, to their detriment." Moreover, the paths from the liver and spleen to the cavity of the thorax are covered by Cimmerian[123] darkness. Hence we are forced to decide that from opened and disrupted vessels and ducts, which are found in the chest, the serous fluid falls into the thoracic cavity and causes this [kind of] dropsy.

In addition to nerves the chest contains blood vessels, lymphatics, and the thoracic duct. We may briefly repeat from the anatomists that this duct, as a cistern or common receptacle of chyle and lymph conveyed from the lower and adjacent parts [of the body], is continued and extended through the length of the thorax, and ends in the subclavian vein. Bartholomaeus Eustachius,[124] an anatomist of very great skill and zeal, in his treatise on the azygous vein, Antigramma 13, calls it the great white—from chyle, of course—off-shoot, full of watery or lymphatic fluid. We owe more exact information to Johannes Pecquetus,[125] to Biepaeus, and others. The lymphatics also with which the pulmonary tunic is invested to a clearly astounding degree lead to the thoracic duct; these lymphatics composed of various islands and anastomoses, with one gland and another intervening, enter that same duct. The intercostal spaces also have their lymphatics but always deposit their lymph, by intermediate glands, in the jugular veins, as was observed by Antonius Nuck,[126] a man who gained great fame in the study of lymphatics, in his anatomical epistle on new discoveries. Nuck even saw the external surface of the heart densely packed with a large number of lymphatics.[127] In fact, since so many lymphatic vessels are found in the thorax, it is not to be doubted that a large multitude of congregated glands is present there. According to the opinion of Malpighi, expressed in a diligent letter dedicated to the Royal Society of England[128] on the structure of the glands and similar structures, the lymphatic vessels are attached to these glands and have close connection with their substance, although the distinguished Nuck, and also Peyer in his Exerci-

tatio 25, page 141,[129] believe that these glands admit lymph and vessels coming from elsewhere rather than emitting them. From the very great assiduity of Ruysch, the prince of the anatomists of our century, we are aware what fate some men fear for the glands; he seems clearly to proscribe all the glands from the body. Nevertheless we consider it right to adhere to the accepted doctrine until experiments more reliable than those which up to the present time have been cited in Ruysch's[130] Problematic Letters shall order us, like soldiers, into his camp.

3. If this is assumed to be true, it is evident that the fluid which is the cause of pectoral dropsy streams out of the nerves in vain; by many recent writers the [existence of] the nerve fluid is utterly rejected. For example Nuck[131] in his treatise on the water channels of the eyes does not hesitate to assert that so far as he knew "no one had succeeded in examining nerve fluid and that when nerves were cut no fluid came forth." And even if this is true, as Malpighi writes on page 39 of his posthumous works,[132] "when the terminal tubules of nerves are cut where they break up into their last subdivisions a juice comes forth"; and "a nerve compounded of three or four tubes," such as is found in the tail of the ox, pours out juice when wounded, which "is fluid and sticky like the sap of the turpentine-tree," nevertheless, before many other things it must be considered that the quantity of this fluid—if there is any at all—is so small that the cavity of the chest cannot be flooded (as usually happens in dropsy of the chest) by it alone. Therefore, it must be that the serous fluid is poured out into the cavity of the chest either from the blood vessels, the lymphatics, or both.

4. But if we recall to memory what kind of fluid is found in persons who have died of dropsy, it is certainly pure and transparent, resembling water in color. Sometimes it is mucilaginous verging on gelatinous, and it will have to be asserted unequivocally that this fluid floods out of the lymphatic vessels into the chest. For it is known from the physiologists that lymph is a pellucid fluid which flows from various membranaceous and muscular structures and glands through transparent and special vessels like aqueducts into the blood. If the vessels themselves are damaged, and this passage is blocked, the fluid falls into the chest, etc.[133] Nor is it unknown to anyone that lymph which has escaped from its

[123] According to ancient legend the Cimmerians, neighbors of the Cumaean sibyl, were cave-dwellers. Hence the use of the adjective to apply to the viscera is completely appropriate. See Tibullus III. V. 24.

[124] Bartholomaeus Eustachius, Opuscula Anatomica (Venice, 1564), antigramma 13, p. 301..

[125] John Pecquet, New Anatomical Experiments (London, 1653), pp. 5 ff.

[126] Antonius Nuck, Adenographia Curiosa et Uteri Foeminei Anatome Nova Cum Epistola ad Amicum de Inventis Novis (Leyden, 1692), pp. 139–152.

[127] Nuck, loc. cit., p. 143.

[128] Marcellus Malpighius, De Structura Glandularum Conglobatarum Consimiliumque Partium. In his Opera Postuma (Amsterdam, 1700), p. 141.

[129] Johann Conrad Peyer, Exercitatio Anatomico-Medica de Glandulis Intestinorum (Schaffhausen, 1677). I have been unable to identify the relevant passage.

[130] Fredericus Ruysch, Opera Omnia (4 v., Amsterdam 1737). The second volume contains many leters designated as "epistolae anatomicae problematicae."

[131] Antonius Nuck, Ductuum Aquosorum Anatome Nova. In his Sialographia (Leyden, 1690), p. 100.

[132] Marcellus Malpighius, Opera Posthuma (London, 1697), p. 27.

[133] In this context et cetera probably means "and elsewhere."

channels congeals like gelatin in the presence of cold and turns into a gelatinous fluid when heat is applied. Spoiled lymph often loses its natural color. Marcellus Donatus[134] observed it to be green and yellow, and Guarinonius[135] found it yellow verging on black. Whenever it stagnates under the skin it is usually found to be ashen gray. That it is occasionally malodorous, like saliva—which assuredly has great affinity with lymph—is evident from the case of the scorbutic citizen of Hamburg, concerning whom consult Dolaeus[136] in *Ephemerid. Dec. Ann.* 9, 10, *Observ.* 131. In section 15 of the preceding chapter we reported that fluid of this kind is found after death in the thoracic cavity of dropsical persons. That the fluid is also sharp, salty, and acid is shown by [the presence of] itching in some dropsical patients and scabies in others. Hence you can understand what the sharp fluid was that Sylvius found in the chest of a young girl.

Indeed it is completely credible that the fluid, having accumulated in excess and finding no outlet in the periphery, by the aid of heat and the helpful delicacy of the structures, drips for the most part by transudation from the lymphatics into the cavity of the chest. Moreover that lymph rushes down into the thoracic cavity even from disrupted glands, we have learned from Bartholinus, who reported in century 2 of his *Anatomical Histories* (History 66)[137] that hydatids, like a fountain, inundated the right side with an abundance of water. Willis[138] confirms this excellently by the example of a young man given to excessive physical exercise, who first "felt a fulness or distention in his chest, so that the left side of his lung seemed to swell and the heart seemed to be pushed out of place." After a period of time he on a certain day "had the feeling that a vessel had burst within the cavity of his chest. For half an hour after this he felt in that region as if there was a dripping of fluid falling from above into the bottom of his chest. The patient himself felt the dripping and it could also be heard by the bystanders." This very thing was also observed by Hippocrates, who said that "water collects in the chest from tubercles which arise there and burst." He shows this by definite evidence in the cow and pig, in his book on internal diseases,[139] using

these words: "I have evidence in the cow, the dog, and the pig, that this happens from tubercles under the skin." Alternatively someone might prefer to maintain that hydatids are lymphatic vessels which, through long-continued distention, have assumed the appearance of bullae or vesicles.

5. Moreover, Willis[140] not unreasonably believes that serum even in its own form[141] exudes into the thoracic cavity, since experience abundantly confirms that "watery weak blood here and there sends out superfluous serum from its structure, and throws it out through lax and patent openings in the arteries, and shuts it out from the texture of the circulation." Therefore it can easily happen that other cavities and also the region of the chest may suffer inundation of this kind.

It is the more probable that dropsy of the chest is sometimes produced in this way since it is quite certain—and has also been observed by ourselves elsewhere—that in subcutaneous structures the blood vessels, damaged neither by cutting nor by puncture, are sometimes opened by disease of the blood or by their own weakness. And although the latter accumulation of serum, caused by disease of the blood or of the blood vessels, is illustrated by the description of hydrocephalics and also through the industry of Wepfer in his learned treatise on the place affected in apoplexy[142]; nevertheless, with respect to the subject under discussion, the fluid that is repeatedly found in the chest after death places such [accumulation] beyond all doubt. Certainly either it is bloody and evidences the source from which it has flowed, or it is similar to the washings of freshly killed meats and again and again offers an indication of its escape from the blood vessels. Unquestionably Charletonius[143] is deceived in thinking that such is the natural color of lymph. Further, this serous afflux happens either through anastomosis,[144] the farthest orifices of the capillary vessels being opened, or through diapedesis in a cacochymic and scorbutic bodily constitution when the blood is so thin and serous that the watery part

---

[134] Marcellus Donatus, *De Medica Historia Mirabili Libri Sex* (Mantua, 1586), book 4, chap. 21, p. 236 *verso*.

[135] Christophorus Guarinonius, *Consilia Medicinalia* (Venice, 1610), consilium 349, pp. 357–358.

[136] J. Dolaeus, "De Vermibus in Saliva," *Miscellanea Curiosa Medico-Physica Academiae Naturae Curiosorum sive Ephemeridum Medico-Physicarum Germanicarum*, [Decuria I], annus IX, obs. 130 (Nuremberg, Endter, 1693), pp. 305–306. This reference given in the Breslau text is defective and inaccurate.

[137] Thomas Bartholinus, *Historiarum Anatomicarum Rariorum Centuria I et II* (Amsterdam, 1654), centuria 2, historia 66, p. 263.

[138] Thomas Willis, *Pharmaceutice Rationalis, Pars Secunda* (London, 1675), sect. 1, chap. 13, p. 229.

[139] Kühn II. 469.

[140] Willis, *op. cit.*, p. 228.

[141] I.e. unaltered.

[142] Johannes Jacobus Wepfer, *Observationes anatomicae, ex cadaveribus eorum, quos sustulit apoplexia* (Schaffhausen, 1658).

[143] Walter Charleton, *Oeconomia Animalis* (London, 1669), p. 211.

[144] These terms are explained in part by a passage in Celsus (IV. 11. 3): Auctores medici sunt vel exesa parte aliqua sanguinem exire, vel rupta, vel ore alicuius venae patefacto: primam διάβρωσιν, secundamρηξιν, tertiam ἀναστόμωσιν appellant. Ultima minime nocet, prima gravissime. This is translated by W. G. Spencer in the Loeb Library edition (1: p. 393) as follows: According to medical authorities blood gains exit either from some part eroded, or ruptured, or from the opened mouth of some blood-vessel; the first they call diabrosis, the second rhexis, the third anastomosis. The last is the least harmful, the first, the worst.

See also Laurentius Bellini, *De Urinis et Pulsibus, de Missione Sanguinis* (Bologna, 1683), pp. 586 *et seq.*

cannot be contained within the hollow of the vessels, or finally through diaeresis [division] and especially diasrosis [separation], disruption, and erosion of continuity, when the entire mass of the blood abounds with sharp and corrosive humors.

But perhaps it is better to admit frankly that the manner in which serum flows out of the blood-vessels and lymphatics cannot be determined accurately and it does not much matter whether the practitioner knows [the facts] or not. Indeed there is no use in pursuing these matters any further, since not so much the urine, tears, sweat, etc. but also certain diseases, such as catarrhs, serous diarrhea, arthritis, and the like, prove how easily serum is separated from blood. Carolus Piso proves this, and adds many other distinct evidences, in his most learned book on the accumulation of serum.[145] Since this happens in the entire body and in all its parts, there is no reason for us not to believe that it also happens in dropsy of the chest.

6. Further, the learned Willis[146] does not doubt that "dropsy of the chest can also be produced by the rupture of chyliferous vessels within the chest." Nevertheless he adds that this happens so rarely that thus far he had never known of it, either from his own observation or from the report of others. And indeed, although it does not happen so often, incontestably the thoracic duct is subject to those ills which cause the rupture of vessels elsewhere. That this duct sometimes is strongly stretched is shown by the squeezing pain which wet-nurses occasionally feel in their backs. This pain perhaps has no other cause than excessive distention of the lacteal vessels and thoracic duct by an abundance of chylous material. This is obvious from the treatment, which is most successfully accomplished by moderation in diet and abstinence from rich foods.

That even the thoracic duct occasionally becomes blocked is easily understood by anyone who accurately weighs the fact that the duct opens into the left subclavian [vein] not by a broad orifice but by six or seven tiny foramina which can easily become obstructed. But whatever the case may be, it is certain that wherever it ultimately arises—whether from lymphatics or blood vessels or even from the thoracic duct—the serous fluid, which we have stated to be the source of dropsy, accumulates not rapidly but gradually. Often a certain quantity of it has been in the chest for a long time; it causes no trouble and moreover gives indistinct signs of its presence. However when, as usually happens, through continual afflux it increases like a torrent and becomes spoiled and quite acrid through stagnation, it necessarily produces dry cough and causes a disturbance of respiration proportionate to its quantity. Finally, when [the fluid] is so pungent that it can no longer be held

within the thoracic cavity, it compresses the lungs and by this compression it suddenly kills the man.

7. The cause of the extravasation of lymph and bloody serum must be sought either in the fluids or in the vessels and viscera, or in all simultaneously. To speak first of the effusion of lymph, it is appropriate to accuse the great thickening of lymph, which prevents the lymph from becoming absorbed by its own [lymphatic] vessels and also by the blood vessels, and from being carried back appropriately to the source of the blood. In the beginning this thickened lymph overwhelms the more delicate pores and channels, distinctly impairs their strength by excessive humidity and predisposes to a solution of continuity. It provides the occasion for rupture, while through stasis it becomes bitter and salty, although a new wave of oncoming lymph always presses upon the old so that either the thicker part of the stagnating lymph, or all of it, is pushed out through the very relaxed pores. Then the lymph becomes rather musty, since it is not properly separated from the salty and fat serum which abounds in musty components in organs dedicated to this secretion and separation, among which the liver has first place and the glandular organs are second. This must necessarily occur, since it is known to everyone from the laws of our very wise Creator that the union between lymph and serum must not be perpetual but the lymph alone, without combination with serum, is carried quietly along in the lymphatic vessels and finally is poured into the vital fluid, so that in the arteries, as if in a marriage bed, it is amicably commingled with the serum.

The aforementioned [process] of separation, as we have already indicated, is delayed especially in the liver when its pores, by which the separation is accomplished, are notably damaged. For this reason various diseases of the liver occasionally are found post mortem in [cases of] ascites and thoracic dropsy, and it is not so very illogical to look in the abdominal cavity for the source of the serous fluid that stagnates in the chest. Moreover this disease increases day by day when the musty dyscrasia of the serum is not cleaned away either by transpiration or urination and is not fluidified. Among the more evident causes of thickening of the lymph not the least important is cold water drunk in abundance when the body is warm; this congeals the serum and lymph. Prosper Martianus,[147] the learned interpreter of Hippocrates, in his discussion of De Morbis, book 2, sect. 3, p. 182 et seq. cites the following statement of Hippocrates from the Book on Internal Diseases, sect. 2, line 76:[148]

Dropsy comes from this: when a person annoyed by thirst in summer drinks much water (for it comes mainly from this) and the lung is filled and discharges again against the chest, etc.

[145] C. Piso, op. cit. (footnote 26).

[146] Willis, op. cit. (footnote 45), sect. 1, chap. 13, p. 232.

[147] Prosper Martianus, Magnus Hippocrates Cous Prosperi Martiani Notationibus Explicatus (Rome, 1626), p. 182.

[148] Kühn II. 469.

This passage Martianus explains as follows: during the very act of swallowing a portion of the drink slips down into the trachea (Hippocrates in his book *On the Heart*, line 14,[149] confirmed this by concrete experience) and "the lungs either because of the quantity of the fluid or because of their own weakness cannot overcome this water. In the course of time the fluid is poured by the lungs into the cavity of the chest, and little by little both the thorax and the lung are filled."

The evaluation of this opinion we leave to others. It should be sufficient for them that Hippocrates elsewhere (in his book *Airs, Waters, and Places*, text XI, p. 338) [150] condemns swamps, standing waters, and lakes as highly fatal sources of dropsy. From other teaching of the same [physician of] Cos we know that cold is unfavorable for the chest. Even cold air does its share. Julius Caesar Benedictus[151] in Consult. 44, p. 185, in discussing the evident causes of the pectoral dropsy from which his brother was suffering, mentions as not irrelevant "a bad way of living and exposure to cold." At the present time in all of Germany and in the metropolis of Silesia many more develop dropsy from drinking aqua vitae, as it is called, than from drinking cold water. The way it is generated is no longer obscure, since the distinguished Boyle[152] in Experiment 8 of his *History of the Blood* cleverly showed that alcoholic spirit of wine when added to the serum of blood changes it into a coagulum or white mass and thus disposes it to stagnation.

8. Not only the fluid lymph but also the very vessels in which it flows can provide the foundation for trouble and in fact do provide it, although the diseases of vessels, except for excessive narrowness in the extremities, are for the most part as yet unknown. The narrowness either is due to natural conformation and origin, or is a product of disease, or is brought on by various compressing and constricting causes, such as inflammatory fluids of various kinds including scirrhous, abnormal concretions around viscera, and the like. Among these causes a place must be given to astringent medicaments, because nowadays everyone knows how easily dropsy appears after fevers have been suppressed, in the fashion of the empirics, by means of strong astringents. There are also cases in which nosebleeds suppressed by strong astringents have given rise to dropsy. Hence it can no longer be doubted that disease of lymphatic vessels often induces dropsy. Carolus Piso acknowledged this and considered it a more frequent cause of dropsy than even dyscrasia of the serum or lymph. It is certain that dropsy arising from disease of the

vessels becomes much more severe in a short time and is very hard to cure. Diseases of vessels are associated with diseases of other organs, which disturb the movement of lymph, and also with diseases of the lungs, which anatomists have found to be impaired by more than one defect in this disease, and have been attacked by induration, scirrhus, and by other swellings and cavities. We have recounted [this] in the preceding chapter. The adherence of lobes of the lung to the pleura, whatever the cause might be, altogether blocks the movement of lymph, although it does not immediately produce dropsy of the chest; we remember that this has been established by several physicians.

With the permission of the reader we may mention here two cases seen by Dr. [Christian] Helwich.[153] A noblewoman of illustrious descent was born in the nearby kingdom of Poland. In the flower of her youth she had scarcely recovered from measles, when, at about Eastertime, she suddenly developed aphonia. A physician was called and came immediately. He prescribed liquor of hartshorn succinate in a potion of water of linden flowers, tunica epileptica,[154] syrup of lavender, and peony flowers. Three hours after she had taken this medicine she spoke pleasantly to those around her but in a short time afterward she lost her speech again and was shaken by horrible convulsions and vomited various substances. Her regular physician being absent, another was called. He opened a vein. A vesicant was applied and excellent remedies were given, all to no effect. On the third day she died. The body was opened. All the abdominal organs were free from disease. When the middle cavity [the chest] was reached, the right lobe of the lung was [found to be] very tightly attached to the pleura. Otherwise the lungs and the heart were in proper condition. Not a drop of fluid was found in the thoracic cavity. In the head the blood vessels were unnaturally distended without any extravasation.

A fifty-year-old man of cholerico-melancholic temperament and still youthful, had chosen a divine and sacred way of life. For more than twenty years he had addressed the public very fervently from the pulpit and had not permitted his diligence in singing the praises of the Lord in chorus to be excelled. For many years there had been no occasion for him to complain of ill health, for he ate with appetite and by drinking wine he would assuage whatever cares he may have had, except that five hours after lunch and seven or eight hours after dinner he would have a tickling in his throat and he was troubled by rather violent cough, which annoyed him for half an hour

---

[149] Kühn II. 485.

[150] Kühn I. 533.

[151] Julius Caesar Benedictus, *Consultationum Medicinalium Opus* (Venice, 1659), consult. 43, p. 185.

[152] Robert Boyle, *Apparatus ad Historiam Naturalem Sanguinis Humani* (Geneva, 1686), p. 24.

[153] See above, footnote 30.

[154] Probably *Cariophyllus hortensis*. According to J. Schröder, *Pharmacopoeia Medico-Chymica* (Ulm, 1649–1650), book 4, p. 38, this plant was also called *tunica* and was used for epilepsy and other nervous diseases.

and in which he brought up viscid and glutinous phlegm in large amounts. He had done everything to banish the hateful sickness from his body. He had used venesection to no avail. In vain he used nodules and other purges and emetics, and he derived no benefit from electuary syrups and sugared potions, which at other times he had liked. Indeed, the sickness increased with the passage of time, and in the autumn of the previous year, as a climax to his afflictions he twice had an intermittent tertian fever, which was broken by merely two or three saline powders and a laxative. He recovered and returned to his duties. About the end of autumn everything went bad again. His cough increased and a hectic fever was added to it. Whatever remedies were used, his strength was very greatly worn away although, as he used to say, on some nights a peaceful sleep of several hours would revive him and in the daytime he would take his food with three or more times greater appetite and quantity than his sickness seemed [able to] tolerate. Later he also had edematous swelling of the feet, his thirst increased, and his expectoration became more difficult day by day. At last, worn out by fever, he gave up his soul to the Creator. The Reverend Father Michael Fibiger, our patron, was pleased to grant permission for the cadaver to be opened and the cause of the illness to be investigated. This was done in the presence of Dr. Christian Helwich and of the most noble Dr. Eggerdes[155] and Dr. Gottofredus Klaunig.[156] The stomach was like paper (so that it was astonishing that it could perform the coction of food ingested in such large amounts) and was empty. The liver was very seriously damaged and dry; it came apart when touched lightly with the fingers. The spleen was marked with black spots. Surprisingly, notable lesions of the mesenteric glands and pancreas could not be seen. When the chest was opened the lung was [found to be] very tightly bound to the ribs but there was no sign of extravasation of lymph or serum, perhaps because by the aid of heat the viscous lymph that had escaped from the vessels had acquired the consistence of little membranes.

9. But we must return from our digression and consider how it happens that the blood sends out serum from the vessels into the cavity of the chest. To extricate the subject from circumlocutions, we cannot fail to recognize disease either in the blood itself, or in the bloodvessels and the viscera connected [to them], or in both at once. As for disease of the blood, although this may be the place for acrimony and deleterious saline power, yet in this harmful function first place is claimed by great viscosity, the cause of obstructions. This viscosity arises from dys-

pepsia[157] on account of raw admixtures and a sluggish menstruum, whatever it may have been; and from unsuitable admixed fluids in the duodenum and in the other coils of intestine, which produce a diseased secretion of chyle from the dregs. We can rightly accuse the transfer of dregs to the blood and the more sluggish movement of the blood and resultant stagnations and inflammations in the viscera, which various [diseased] conditions of the viscera produce, etc. Space does not allow us to enumerate here the harmful actions of unnatural foods and components in [producing] this result. However, we cannot conceal the harmfulness of aqua vitae, since the distinguished Bohnius[158] in the *Acta Eruditorum Lipsiensium* for April, 1683, pp. 153 *et seqq.* has demonstrated by clear experiment that the spirit of wine coagulates blood. Before all else it must be noted that impaired movement of lymph or its effusion into any cavity strongly increases the viscosity of the blood and favors stagnation in the bloodvessels. It is established by reason and experience that venous blood is ten times thicker than arterial blood, since the arteries contain ten times more lymph than the veins. It would therefore be necessary for the blood within the veins to be diluted in order to flow back into the heart. For this purpose God the foreseeing maker of the world arranged that the lymphatic vessels flow together into an inferior and superior trunk. But if the movement of lymph is delayed or this lymphatic fluid because of effusion into some cavity is not conveyed into the venous blood, the latter, through lack of dilution will necessarily be too thick. The thickness will cause other sicknesses and also stagnation and obstruction; obviously it must be undone lest it work against the circulation of the blood. Moreover, by such obstruction the viscera are constrained and compressed, and lose their original weight. The same happens in glands, which sometimes waste away and become shriveled when obstructed. Even the lungs, although previously large and wide often become so wasted and narrowed that they are difficult even for physicians to recognize; this can also be said of the obstructed liver and spleen.

When the blood vessels are confined in a narrow space so that they do not allow free passage for the blood, it is impossible for the serum not to be poured forth separately from the blood. This is obvious from the experiment of the eminent Lower.[159] Since they marvelously illustrate the problem under discussion, we shall borrow a few statements from the second

[155] Alardus Mauritius Eggerdes, author of several works on plague and other clincial papers.

[156] Gottfried Klaunig (1676–1731), imperial physician, Stadtarzt at Breslau.

[157] Dyspepsia (literally, bad cooking) is approximately equal to faulty metabolism or metabolic error.

[158] J. Bohn, "Observatio atque Experimenta Circa Usum Spiritus Vini Externum." In *Acta Eruditorum Anno MDCLXXXIII Publicata* (Leipzig, 1683), pp. 153–156.

[159] Richardus Lower, *Tractatus de Corde* (Amsterdam, 1669), p. 124.

chapter of his learned work *On the Heart*, specifically from the passage on page 82 concerning the movement and color of the blood: "Not long ago," he says, "I had tightly tied the jugular veins in a dog by drawing a thread around them. A few hours later all the parts above the ligature were remarkably swollen. Within two days the dog died as if choked by angina.[160] All this while, not only did tears flow very copiously but the animal also salivated abundantly, just as if the flow had been produced by the taking of mercury. After the death of the dog I separated its skin from the swollen parts. I expected that the latter would be distended with extravasated blood, but [the experiment] turned out altogether differently. I could observe no trace or color of blood, but all the muscles and glands appeared very greatly distended by clear serum and quite transparent. This clearly proves that serum somehow is secreted by constriction of veins."

These and other facts referring to our subject Lower has placed on the aforementioned and subsequent pages [of his book]. And on this principle, while we investigate the causes of viscidity of the serum, we know at the same time in what way the blood vessels themselves combine their effects, both with the lymphatic vessels and the blood, to bring about the outpouring of serum, while both the blood vessels and the organs connected with them are stuffed with glutinous blood. This usually happens in dropsy of the chest, as is shown by the example of the man whose case we have already cited from the writing of Blanckardus,[161] who expressly states on page 265 that at the beginning of the great artery [aorta] there were certain little hillocks of blood and to this grumous blood the same author attributes the deficiency in the pulse which he had previously observed.

10. It is not in this way alone, which we have already discussed, that the very vessels in which the blood is carried cause a delay in the movement of the blood and dispose to stagnation and dropsical outpouring of serum. In many other ways, while they are being dilated or shortened, etc. certainly in a peculiar manner the ossification of the vessels acts to this effect, as we have stated in chapter I. Because of bony[162] protuberances and irregularities the arteries doubtless lose their power of expanding and dilating. The autopsy of Wepfer shows that blood was dashed against them (as against rocks) and was accumulated within the precordia and that lymph finally flowed out. The importance of the subject requires that we again excerpt some passages from his history and that

we explain in the words of Brunner what the condition of his arteries was. Brunner on page 163 of the work previously cited[163] writes the following:

The aorta behind the semilunar valves repelled the inserted fingers with a bony roughness and a certain sharp prominence pricked them. In its course it was found to be wholly made up of cartilaginous semicircles, at least indurated if not altogether bony, as far as the bifurcation of the iliac arteries. Near the renal arteries a distinctly bony circle one inch broad surrounded the aorta. The farther from the heart the more the aorta was found to be bony, especially near the iliacs, which retained their bony hardness when torn away from the thighs. Finally I freed the aorta from its integuments and carefully cleaned it in order to examine it deeply. Indeed I cut into it forcefully with scissors in order to observe its inner parts. On the inside its natural whiteness and smoothness were missing and the channel for the blood although not completely cut off was scurfy, shaggy, and rugged, and the internal coat was roughened by various irregularities and bony protuberances about the origin of the coeliac, and below the renals it was disrupted.

It is certain that this kind of ossification of vessels is also found in other bodies. The following comments of Lucius[164] are pertinent:

In the body (of a melancholic old man) the cardiac arteries were found to be bony within the heart. They had hardened, as commonly happens in the hearts of the aged and also of beasts, and very often in the hearts of deer.

Whoever considers this will scarcely regard as a wondrous miracle of nature the chariot [made] from "the ribs of oxen of which the entire overlying flesh had turned into completely genuine bone." This is kept in a museum by the eminent Master Rosenringe with the observations of Bircherod, as can be read in the *Literary News of the Baltic* for the year 1705, p. 221.[165]

There is no doubt that a polypous or any other concretion with ossified vessels can be responsible for the same effect. It is known that in the dilated great artery [aorta] of the distinguished Charles Patin this kind of body was found, "larger than a big goose egg and weighing three or four ounces. In shape it resembled the fruit of a thistle." In this way it is described in detail in the extraordinary *Medical Letter on Polyp of the Aorta* in the appendix to year I, decuria III, p. 116 [of the *Ephemerides*].[166] Indeed in the same letter it is clear that the feet "were affected by edematous swelling." Hence it can be understood by easy conjecture how greatly impediments of this kind in the vessels disturb the movement

---

[160] Angina, formerly used for various kinds of swelling of the throat, usually caused by infection.

[161] S. Blancard, *Anatomia Practica Rationalis* (Amsterdam, 1688), centuria 2, obs. 48, p. 265.

[162] anatomists of this era used the term *osseus* (bony) to refer to sclerotic plaques and especially calcifications not necessarily converted into true bone.

[163] J. Brunner, *op. cit.* (footnote 39), p. 163.

[164] D. I. G. Lucius, "Observatio Medica de Glandula Pineali Petrefacta et Osse in Corde Reperto," *Nova Literaria Germaniae* (Hamburg, 1705), p. 254.

[165] *Nova Literaria Maris Balthici et Septentrionis* (Lübeck, 1705), p. 221.

[166] A. Knipsmacoppe, *"De Aortae Polypo Epistola Medica,"* *Ephemeridum Medico-Physicarum Germanicarum Academiae Caesareo-Leopoldinae Naturae Curiosorum*, Decuriae III, Annus Primus, appendix p. 116 (Leipzig, 1694).

of the blood and contribute to the accumulation of serum in parts [of the body]. When the movement of the blood is turned askew even hematosis,[167] which owes its origins to the internal and periodic movement of blood, is weakened. Less valuable blood, unsuitable for nutrition, is produced. This supplies a fresh cause for the origin of dropsy.

11. Finally, it is exceedingly easy to understand in what manner and as a result of what causes chyle can be poured out of the thoracic duct and by such outpouring can produce a flood in the chest and can cause and hasten death. Two experiments of Lower, described in his aforementioned book[168] (chap. 5, p. 154 *et seq.*), make this matter very clear. This distinguished man opened the chest of a dog on the right side between two lower ribs. He inserted his finger and having cut his fingernail to resemble a saw, he cut through and tore the common receptacle,[169] which was greatly distended three hours after the animal had eaten. After this had been done and the wound had been sewn together, he fed the animal to satiety. Within a few days the dog died and he put it under the anatomist's knife. He found the stomach and intestines very full and indeed the lacteal vessels also were filled with chyle. In that side of the chest in which the common receptacle had been opened he found two pounds of chyle. He tried the same experiment in another dog. Making a hole in the left side between the third and fourth ribs, he inserted his finger through the opening of the wound and broke the duct. As before, he stuffed the dog [with food]. A short time afterward, when it not only weakened but died, he dissected the chest of this animal likewise. That chamber of the chest in which the duct had been disrupted was completely filled with chyle and the lung was stuck to that side. Indeed, in the judgment of Willis,[170]

it is of no importance to look into the etiology of this disease, which is not only incurable but also rapidly fatal, because obviously the precordia are immediately overwhelmed by inundation of chyle and at the same time the blood and the animal spirits, nutritive fluids deprived of their customary tribute, are thereby released.

From these statements it appears that Willis no less than Lower was of the opinion that chyle does not flow into the mesenteric veins from any region. In order to test this, Lower did the experiment which we have cited. Whether or not these entirely end the controversy is still under adjudication, yet it is entirely probable that thoracic dropsy originating from rupture of the thoracic duct cannot fail to throttle a man in a short time.

12. Incontrovertibly, dropsy of the pericardium is produced in the same way, except that the motion of the heart—damaged by disease and fault of the heart itself, or damaged by disease of the containing structures—contributes to the production of pericardial dropsy in an especially stronger manner than defects of the blood and lymph, although the water in the pericardium, accumulated in a larger amount than is appropriate, compresses even the sides of the heart by reason of its weight. Consequently the heart cannot dilate sufficiently to take up [incoming] blood. Zellerus' case, discussed in the last section of chapter I,[171] shows very clearly which diseases afflict the glands and the lymph in this malady. For the lentil-sized granules with which the pericardium of the soldier was bestrewn and roughened cannot be considered to be anything else than tiny glands which in the natural condition elude the keenness of the eye and even of the microscope. Colloquially they are called miliary. In this diseased subject they had grown to that size. They have the same fate in other parts of the body also. Thus we remember that in the inner coat of the stomach these glands have been seen to be as large as small filberts.

In the great obscurity of this subject it is most unprofitable to submit many assertions as if they were true or to cling to various conjectures and fabrications which will disappear in time. Therefore no one expects from us that we should decide whether water drips from the pericardium into the chest through concealed ducts or goes frequently from the chest into the pericardium, although the first of these opinions appears to us to be by far the more likely. In solitary dropsy of the lungs the distinguished Tozzius[172] (page 310 of the work already cited) suspects that "in the course of time the pores and vesicles of the lung are filled with lymph which has become stickier in that place and is not conveyed through its own channels; indeed the fumes are concreted by some acid" or, impeded in some such manner, "stuff the substance of the lungs and provoke dropsy." "Not rarely," says Tozzius, "it even happens that hydatids grow on to the lungs from watery fluid that distends the outermost [pulmonary] membrane, which at some point is relaxed. By common opinion, which follows the teaching of Hippocrates in his book *On Internal Diseases*,[173] these vesicles, filled with water, are thought to accompany dropsy [of the chest]."

13. Some visceral ailments, which we have cataloged near the end of chapter I, are so connected in this disease that they combine like causes in the production of dropsy; with others, indeed, the condition is such that they must be reckoned among the effects and products of dropsy.

In the first of these two categories, as we have already indicated several times in previous [pages],

---

[167] The formation of new blood.
[168] Lower, *op. cit.* (footnote 159), chap. 5, pp. 219–222.
[169] The receptaculum chyli.
[170] Willis (*op. cit.*, footnote 45), chap. 13, p. 232.

[171] Zellerus' case is discussed in chap. I, sect. 17, above.
[172] Tozzius, *op. cit.* (footnote 101), p. 237.
[173] Kühn II. 429.

we have placed the more important diseases of the filtering organs and various corruptions of the liver, spleen, lungs, etc. As for the kidneys you may justifiably doubt whether their obvious degeneration in persons who have died of this disease are not rather to be regarded as some [kind of] morbid product. Diseases of the lungs, which participate in the generation of this disease more effectively than diseases of other organs, if you consider the matter accurately, almost all derive from a very copious congestion of the blood [which goes] to the lungs, for from this source haemoptysis streams forth and also the ulcerations that are so closely allied [to haemoptysis] in the bloodless condition of this organ. Or if perchance blood does not burst forth, by this very congestion the opportunity is afforded for dry cough, periodic asthma, various irritations, pressures, stagnations, and for the inflammations which arise from these sources, as well as their consequences—abscesses of more than one kind, cavities and other erosions and ruptures of lymphatic vessels, etc. Therefore dropsy of the chest is quite well known in that time of life which is susceptible to congestions of blood in the region of the chest.

In the second category we place thickening of the membranes which encircle the chest—doubtless this arises from prolonged stagnation of water in that place—and also various deteriorations of bile, which result either from a moldy composition of the serous fluids or from disease of the liver, etc.

14. We shall not tarry long to recount the remoter causes of this disease.[174] It is commonly known that persons of phlegmatic and sanguineous temperament are subject to every kind of dropsy, including the kind that is under discussion here. This is true also of those who subsist on the thicker foods, from which viscid blood and chyle originate. Previously, when discussing what causes lymph to thicken, we rightly condemned unhealthful drinks, such as water prepared from melted snow, cold potions [taken in] summertime, etc. Nor do we hesitate to include in this list beer made from grain, especially when it is fresh, insufficiently cleared of sediment, or badly prepared. In the causation of dropsy a role must also be assigned to thick cloudy air, which is seen plainly enough in swampy and maritime places where dropsy is quite common.[175] Toward the accumulation of serum in quantity, even excessive sleep is contributory, also idleness, to say nothing of affections of the mind; among the latter many [writers] point to sadness, anger, and sudden fright. More powerful causes are suppression and retention of excretions.

Concerning poison there is a question whether it must be accorded a place among the causes of pectoral dropsy. In chapter I we stated that Maximilian II, the love and delight of the human race, died of pectoral dropsy, and some suspicion of poisoning arose among the most famous physicians of that time. It is rumored that Hercules Saxonia publicly asserted in lectures given in Padua that "this extremely gentle emperor had been carried off by poison." Bertius[176] in book II of the *German Commentaries* reports that "it was administered to him by Granvellanus and to such a degree that Maximilian suffered for twenty entire years from palpitation of the heart." Of the same opinion was Hieronymus Mercurialis,[177] an absolutely outstanding physician. In the first volume of his *Medical Consultation* 111, p. 257, he wrote expressely as follows: "Consequently I judge that the origin of all the trouble was poison ingested in birds and in mushrooms." But the reasons which he gives are not compelling. For when he could not otherwise discover the cause of the various symptoms that troubled the Emperor, this distinguished physician alone relied upon the excellent bodily constitution which His Majesty had had in his youth; and by some unknown process of reasoning, since the symptoms did not conspire to create that world of troubles, he infers that the ruler had been poisoned, whereas he should have inferred instead that plethora had caused both the dropsy and the other sickness. Apart from this it cannot be denied that those slow poisons (which several men believe to be prepared from sugar of lead by the addition of a certain more volatile corrosive) very unobtrusively and gradually throw men into cachexia and dropsy.

The diseases which this [pectoral] dropsy follows are various. The chief among them are scurvy, asthma, and dysentery, [also] haemoptysis and other diseases of the chest. From this it is evident that pectoral dropsy attacks mainly youths and persons established in maturity. It afflicts infants rather rarely. The eminent Harderus reported in his *Apiarium* (Beehive)[178] the case of a rather fat boy in whom in addition to other things he found, "a thin bloody replica of a spider web, partly destroyed, and lungs dripping with serous and foamy fluid, [and] an abundance of waters moving about in the cavity of the chest." And Dr. Pauli[179] took care of a noble boy who during life could never tolerate a cincture about his chest. When this patient died in convulsions he

---

[174] I.e. dropsy of the chest.

[175] Possibly a reference to the dropsy which may occur in quartan malaria.

[176] Petrus Bertius, *Commentariorum Rerum Germanicarum* (Amsterdam, 1616), p. 263.

[177] Hieronymus Mercurialis, *Responsorum et Consultationum Medicinalium, Tomus Primus* (Venice, 1587), consult. 111, p. 257.

[178] J. J. Harderus, *Apiarium* (Basel, 1689), obs. 51 (scholium), p. 218. Harder's text reads "omentum tenue instar aranearum telae," the thin omentum, like a spider web. This the Breslau authors, no doubt accidentally, altered to "cruentum tenue instar . . ."

[179] Probably either Johannes Guilielmus Pauli (1658–1723) professor in the medical faculty at Leipzig or Michael Pauli (1652–?), Stadtarzt at Breslau.

was found to have both sides of his chest filled with blackish water.

Now an account must be given of the principal symptoms [of pectoral dropsy].

15. Distress and oppressive pain in the precordium offer an indication of serum contained in some place outside the vessels and distending the fibers. That such tensions of fibers may arise from serum effused even in no great quantity is evident from the feet of ascitic persons, who complain of the distention even when no noteworthy swelling of the feet is present. On what the difficulty of breathing in pectoral dropsy depends cannot be explained more accurately than if we present in a few words [taken] from the physiologists the manner in which the reciprocal movement of the ribs produces dilatation and contraction of the thorax. It is true that Thomas Bartholinus[180] in his *Anatomia Reformata* insists that the ribs are raised by the external intercostal muscles and by constriction of the chest subserve expiration, whereas they are brought together by the internal [intercostal muscles] and by dilatation they aid inspiration. Spigelius[181] indeed (book IV, chap. 8), with many followers, believes [the chest] is dilated and contracted in this act. We, however, think it preferable to stick to the opinion of Plempius,[182] Sylvius,[183] Schwammerdamm,[184] and the learned Mayow.[185] The last-named, by arguments based on mechanics and on the very conformation and articulation of the ribs, has made it probable that the costal arch is not moved outward in inspiration and inward in expiration; instead, it is drawn upward and downward. In the former process when [the arch] is drawn upward the space in the chest is dilated; in the latter, while [the arch] is drawn downward the chest is contracted. At the very moment in which the ribs are elevated and the chest is raised, the diaphragm exchanges its convexity, which faces the abdomen, for flatness, so that with mighty force it strikes strongly against the hand. In a word: while it contracts in inspiration it moves away from the cavity of the chest, which it allows to become longer, and it lowers the bottom of the chest. Contrariwise, in expiration, when it relaxes from its contraction it fills the chest again[186] by means of its curvature and it shortens the thoracic cavity. This is explained more

fully by Spigelius, Bartholinus, Sylvius, Schwammerdamm, Mayow, Diemerbroeck,[187] and by Laurentius[188] himself, whose opinion Diemerbroeck seems not to have followed. If we apply these facts to the subject under discussion, it immediately becomes apparent that when expiration must occur, the weight of the water which lies upon the diaphragm hinders it to some extent from filling the cavity of the chest by its [muscular] curvature. Hence it must necessarily result that our dropsical patients breathe in inspiration in the same way that Brunner learnedly observed in the case of his father-in-law [Wepfer].

But what is the reason that the asthmatic affection threatens our patients mainly after the first sleep? Willis[189] believed that this happens on account of "fumes which rise at that time because of more intense heat," and he attributes the great restlessness and jactitation to those same vapors. We have established by experience that this restlessness frequently joined with asthma is usually at its height five hours after dinner. When we reflect that the stomach is emptied for the most part by the fourth hour after dinner, yet the chyle ordinarily does not fully enter the lacteal vessels before the sixth hour, as the eminent Lister not unjustifiably believes (page 152 of his *Comments on the Medical Statics of Sanctorius*),[190] the restlessness is perhaps not unreasonably ascribed in part to chyle that flows into the sea of blood but does not properly mix with it. Further, it is certain that in wakeful persons the muscles are, so to speak, tense and contracted. From this condition of the muscles the narrowness and constriction of the lymphatic glands and vessels certainly arises, most especially in the feet and about the hips, where the glands are especially numerous and large. Moreover, during sleep not only the muscles but also the contracted glands and even the vessels are relaxed, if we believe the statement of Lister (on page 142 of the work already cited) that "he who is awake has all the muscles of his body in a state of contraction and his glandular orifices are twice as narrow as in him who sleeps." If this is true, it is probable that during sleep, while the glands and the orifices of the lymphatic channels are relaxed, there is greater flow [of lymph] to the chest, as if to an injured region, and a greater pressure arises against the lungs from the fluids which flow thither, and the breath is more greatly impeded.

16. The unequal pulse, interrupted now and then, arises from some impediment in the precordia and

[180] Thomas Bartholinus, *Anatomia Reformata* (Leyden, 1651), book 2, chap. 2, pp. 216–217.

[181] Adrianus Spigelius, *De Humani Corporis Fabrica* (Venice, 1627), book 4, chap. 8, pp. 109–116 (esp. pp. 113 ff.).

[182] Vopiscus Fortunatus Plempius, *Fundamenta Medicinae, Edito Tertia* (Louvain, 1654), pp. 133–134.

[183] Franciscus Sylvius, *Opera Medica* (Amsterdam, 1580), p. 889.

[184] J. Schwammerdam, *Tractatus Physico-Anatomico-Medicus de Respiratione Usque Pulmonum* (Leyden, 1667), pp. 14–19.

[185] Johannes Mayow, *Opera Omnia Medico-Physica* (Hague, 1681), pp. 243 ff.

[186] The diaphragm in this phase "fills the chest" not with air but with its own mass.

[187] Isbrandus Diemerbroeck, *Anatome Corporis Humani* (Utrecht, 1672), book 2, chap. 3, p. 423.

[188] Andreas Laurentius, *Historia Anatomica Humani Corporis* (Frankfurt, 1600), book 9, chap. 4, p. 343; book 9, chap. 22, p. 369.

[189] Willis, *op. cit.* (footnote 45), sect. 1, chap. 13, p. 232.

[190] Sanctorius Sanctorius, *De Statica medicina aphorismorum sectiones septem: cum commentario Martini Lister* (London, 1701), §§28 and 29, p. 152.

from the disturbed movement of the fluids which flow from that region. It is quite well known that the pulse or reciprocal outward and inward movement of the arteries, or, as others please to call it, the diastole and systole of the arteries, depend on the systole and diastole of the heart. It is no longer unknown even to beginners in our art that the heart is a muscle which by perpetual alternation receives and expels blood.[191] During its contraction, while its walls come together from all sides, its chambers eject all their blood and become empty, and are filled during relaxation. The pulsations of the arteries correspond to the vibrations of the heart; and the pulse is equal [regular] when the alternating contraction of the heart pushes the blood into the arteries with equal force and in equal amounts within equal intervals of time. Necessarily, therefore, the pulse is unequal [in disease] either because there is a delay in the heart or because an obstacle arises in the influx and efflux of blood or in the movement of fluids. That this very thing occurs in our dropsy [i.e. in dropsy of the chest], is evident from what has already been said. When the lymph flows out again into the cavity of the chest and neither chyle nor blood is appropriately diluted [by it], the result can scarcely be otherwise than that the ventricles of the heart and the blood vessels become enveloped and almost filled by thick fluids, while, like gelatin, they gradually become agglomerated on the walls of the cardiac ventricles and the vessels. That a weak and intermittent pulse arises from this cause is the testimony of Lower in his book, previously cited. Palpitation of the heart, produced in our disease by abundance of water in the pericardium, also arises from these same causes, as Tulpius[192] reports in his Medical Observations, book II, chap. 26 [and also] Carolus Piso in the eleventh chapter[193] of his frequently cited book, likewise Riolanus and many others, not to mention Diemerbroeck,[194] who writes as follows on page 430 of the work already cited:

I have noticed that an [abnormally] large amount of this (pericardial) fluid does not produce palpitation of the heart, although physicians commonly hold a contrary opinion which follows Galen. For in all those in whom I have found a large amount of this watery fluid in the pericardium after death, I found no palpitation whatever during the antecedent illness, but on the contrary the pulse was sluggish and quite slow. Moreover, the excess of this fluid does not produce such oppression of the pericardium that the heart cannot move freely within it and hence palpitates; on the contrary I have always noticed that the pericardium becomes so broad and loose that the heart can move in it more freely than when the fluid is scanty.

We rightly wonder that the fact has escaped this distinguished man, since it is very easy to understand in what way an excessive quantity of water in the pericardium could impede the contractions and dilatations of the heart if it presses by its weight or ferments and swells. Compare Bellini on diseases of the chest on page 616 of his Works.[195]

Not to be rashly derided are the complaints of the sick whose heart palpitates or trembles or moves in a disorderly way, when they say their heart [feels] as if it were swimming in water, when that sensation is much more certain than all the guesses of even the most expert physicians.[196] For this reason when that noble sexagenarian two years previously "had begun to feel a weight in his chest and a certain time afterward also had a kind of tremulous and disorderly movement of the heart, and felt as if his heart were swimming in water," the eminent Raymundus Joannes Fortis[197] (centuria 2, consult. 46, p. 181) correctly inferred that "watery matter had collected in the pericardium." Nor did Hercules Saxonia,[198] in book 2 of the Medicina Practica, chapter 8, p. 179, disbelieve one Galenus of the household of Marcellus, who suffered from this disease (water in the pericardium) together with dropsy of the lung, and before his death became leucophlegmatic. This man said he felt that his heart was swimming in water. We shall not insist on the unanimous agreement of physicians who have noticed palpitation [derived] from an excessive quantity of fluid in the pericardium. Not the last among them are Galen[199] and his followers Fuchsius,[200] Hollerius,[201] Amatus Lusitanus,[202] and many others. And so there is no doubt that dropsy of the chest, just as [happens with] pus in empyema, which pushes the external surface of the pericardium inward, causes palpitation of the heart; and the causes may be fluids, abscesses, grumous blood, etc., as Hollerius somewhere correctly observes.

17. Sebizius believed (p. 892)[203] that fainting is the progeny of vicious and rank vapors which come from

[191] This statement reminds us that the work of Harvey was less than a century old.

[192] Nicolaes Tulp, Observationes Medicae, Editio Nova (Amsterdam, 1652), book 4, chap. 19, pp. 325–327.

[193] Carolus Piso, op. cit. (footnote 26), sect. 3, chap. 2, p. 192.

[194] Diemerbroeck, op. cit. (footnote 187), p. 430.

[195] Laurentius Bellini, Opera Omnia (2nd ed., Venice, 1732) 1: pp. 455 et seq.

[196] Note the high value which the authors wisely place on the patients' statements.

[197] Raymundus Joannes Fortis, Consultationum et Responsionum Medicinalium Centuriae Quattuor (Geneva, 1677), centuria 2, consult. 46, p. 181.

[198] Hercules Saxonia, Pantheum Medicinae Selectum, sive Medicinae Practicae Templum (Frankfurt, 1603), book 2, chap. 8, p. 179.

[199] Galen, De Locis Affectis, book 5, chap. 2. Kühn, VIII. 303.

[200] Leonhardus Fuchsius, De Medendis Singularum Humani Corporis Partium (Basel, 1539), pp. 109–110.

[201] Jacobus Hollerius Stempanus, De Morborum Internorum Curatione (Venice, 1572), book 1, chap. 27, pp. 75 verso–76 recto.

[202] Amatus Lusitanus, Curationum Medicinalium (Venice, 1566), centuria 3, curatio 43, 1: pp. 481–484.

[203] Melchior Sebizius [jun.], Manualis, sive Speculi Medicinae Practici (Argentorati, 1661), part 3, sect. 3, chap. 13, 1: p. 892.

putrid serum and infest the heart. Duretus[204] in the *Coan Prenotions*, p. 131, judges [the matter] more correctly and writes that "by lipopsychia or (incorrectly expressed) lipothymia, is meant a weakness of the animal faculty, analogous to amaurosis of the eyes." What might be the cause of the swooning he does not disclose. Doubtless he does not recognize other causes than that very palpitation of the heart, since it is distinctly established by the cases which the eminent Bonetus[205] collected in his *Anatom[ia] Pract[ica]*, book 2, sect. 10, that some were seized with fainting "because of abscesses which arose either within the substance of the heart or elsewhere"; others "because of stinking fluid enclosed within the ventricle of the heart or in the thoracic cavity"; others "because of a certain polypous concretion," certainly because in this way the movement of fluids is impeded, when some very large and important vessel about the heart is strongly obstructed and the blood is denied free passage, for then it is necessary for forces to be released to a sufficient extent until the obstruction or other impediment to the advance of the compactly onrushing blood may be removed. Moreover our dropsical patients, who quite often are forsaken by consciousness, have the same fate as others who suffer from fainting, without manifest cause: indisputably, in accordance with Hippocratic aphorism,[206] they die suddenly.

18. It has become apparent that cough arises from acrid fluid which stimulates and irritates the diaphragm, the lung, and its vessels, especially if we accept the patients' opinion that the fluid which causes uneasiness in the chest can be torn out through the trachea and removed by way of the throat. Indeed the cough grows powerful when the lung is being very strongly irritated by the water that ferments in the chest. This also happens when the serous collection in the chest is shaken by movement or inappropriate posture of the body. Swellings, if such are present, arise from serum that has escaped from its vessels, unless perchance with other doctors you prefer to blame pituitous [phlegmatic] blood, which produces both swelling and lurid color in the faces of cachectic persons.

Harmony between the chest and the pudenda is certain; it has been observed by Hippocrates and often by others. You will read in Hippocrates, *Epidemics*, book 2, sect. 5,[207] that a dry cough is often relieved by severe pain that invades the testicles;

and in book 2, section 1 of the *Epidemics*,[208] that if cough supervenes on inflammation of the testes, the inflammation is resolved. To the same topic the passage in book 2 of *Prognostics*,[209] 67 etc. is relevant.

It is commonly known that the voice becomes heavier and gradually approaches virile quality at the age when hairs grow at the pubes. It is known further that purulent matter enclosed in the cavity of the chest may be discharged through the urinary passages. Indeed, in Scultetus' *Armamentarium Chirurgicum*, obs. 46 and 51 [210] and in Diemerbroeck, book 1, chap. 17 [211] and in many other writings there is no lack of cases in which pus has been emitted by this route[212] and empyema has been cured. However the facts may be regarded, it is nevertheless extremely difficult to show on what this harmony may be based, unless perchance we are willing to believe with Laurentius in his *Historia Anatomica*, book 9, question 2,[213] that the flood in the chest is carried back to the heart through the veins and is then transferred through the arteries to the kidneys and also to the pudenda. Yet the question still remains why the accumulation in the chest is not carried through the arteries to other parts of the body as much as to the scrotum. We do not know whether those [physicians] extricate themselves more satisfactorily [from the difficulties] who judge that attention should be directed not so much toward any of the bodily channels as toward the lymph which is derived from them and stagnates in [this] condition of the body; and they contend that the culprit is gravitational movement of lymph to the lower structures. For there are no obvious signs of lymph stagnating in the periphery of the body at the time when serous accumulation causes the scrotum to swell. That this harmony depends on special movements might perhaps be evidenced by persons afflicted with cough, in whom it was first noted by Hippocrates.

19. Fever attacks some persons [who have pectoral dropsy]; others indeed are free from it. Without doubt fever afflicts those whose viscera are either obstructed or inflamed or misshapen by some other quite severe disease such as ulcers and abscesses. There is no disputing that persons whose organs are in this condition have fever. As we have already noted, dissection has adequately ascertained that dropsical persons occasionally suffer from such disease of the viscera. Indeed, it is clearly established that these diseases of the organs sometimes are the cause of dropsy. And lest any doubt perchance remain about inflammation, here—albeit out of context—we

---

[204] Ludovicus Duretus, *Hippocratis Magni Coacae Praenotiones* (Paris, 1588), p. 131.

[205] Theophilus Bonetus, *Sepulchretum* (Geneva, 1679). Book 2, sect. 10, pp. 678–692 is titled *De Leipothymia, Syncope*. Obs. 17, p. 685 discusses abscess in the diaphragm; obs. 18, pp. 686–688 discusses pancreatic abscess; obs. 25, p. 690 discusses ruptured intra-abdominal abscess.

[206] Kühn III. 717.

[207] Kühn III. 461.

[208] Kühn III. 461.

[209] Kühn I. 190.

[210] J. Scultetus, *Cheiroplotheke, seu Armamentarium Chirurgicum* (Ulm, 1655), pp. 100 and 103.

[211] Diemerbroeck, *op. cit.* (footnote 187), p. 172.

[212] Through the urinary tract.

[213] Laurentius, *op. cit.* (footnote 23), book 9, question 12, pp. 362–363.

may note what Guarinonius[214] reports in his *Consilia*, no. 349; he had quite often seen inflammation of the lungs fill the chest with water.

That paralysis of the arms comes from compression of blood vessels rather than of nerves, although the latter also contribute to it, is the more probable the more certainly it is established that the ligation of arteries is followed by inability to move; both Steno[215] and Brunner have correctly noted this. The latter,[216] as you can read in Decuria 3 of the *Ephemerides*, years 5 and 6, obs. 293, p. 660, after he had carefully tied the trunk of the descending aorta in a dog, had replaced the intestines, and had sewn the abdominal wound by a few sutures, saw that "the dog was weak and scarcely stood on its feet. Soon it rested on its forelegs and could hardly move its hind legs. Soon they were paralyzed and the dog dragged them along after it." And when Brunner had loosened the binders from the abdomen and had also removed the thread by which the aorta had been constricted, little by little the dog recovered. "First it stood on its forelegs. Presently it moved its hind legs, and finally stood on them and walked as before." Brunner says he learned from this that the experiment is correct by which it is alleged that when the artery [aorta] is tied, movement of the hind legs is abolished.

From these considerations it can be concluded that Riverius[217] is greatly in error when he teaches in book 7, chapter 5, page 255 of his *Practice*, already cited, that the paralysis [that accompanies dropsy] "is caused either by fluid slipping down from the head into the chest, a portion of it flowing into the nearby arm; or by serum contained in the chest and exuding by way of the axillary veins into the arms"; or "by cooling of the intercostal muscles from which the nerves arise that go to the arms" or by "some other related principle." On the other hand Hippocrates, whom Riverius incorrectly cites in his own support, states the contrary in the *Coan* [*Prenotions*] when he derives this kind of paralysis from "violent inflammation of the lungs or pleura" which induces compression of vessels.

20. In our dropsical patients the external structures are cold, because when the circulation of blood is disturbed by the influx of the liquid which is the hearth of all the heat in the body, they undergo deprivation, while the internal organs are burned by intense heat on account of the regurgitating blood. In these patients the appetite is intact because they

have no fever and the stomach is not packed with mucoid or vaporous crudity. They also do not suffer from thirst, since the movement of lymph to the glands in the throat and stomach is not entirely interrupted. However, some dropsical persons, because the movement of lymph to these parts is altogether broken off, are very severely oppressed by intense thirst, which tortures the body more harshly than any pain, as Pechlin correctly observes in the third book of his *Observations*.[218] Food ingested by our dropsical patients in slightly large amounts provokes an asthmatic paroxysm, especially near the end of coction. [This happens] when the stomach is full and is burdened with foodstuffs swollen by foamy fermentation, the movement of the diaphragm, previously impeded, is clogged more and more. As Hercules Saxonia[219] has correctly stated, page 152, "when food is ingested the difficulties are increased, obviously because of pressure made by the full stomach about the diaphragm." Alternatively [postprandial asthma] may arise because new chyle carried to the chest through the thoracic duct, its ordinary channel, increases the compression of the lungs by its weight. Moreover, that asthma occasionally arises from the stomach being excessively distended by food can be observed every day in gluttonous boys. The belly also responds: sometimes because there is no inherent disease in the intestines and they are neither compressed nor inflamed and peristaltic motion is not perverted, and sometimes—that which is the cause of the disturbance—the movement of serum and lymph is obviously not destroyed, hence the excreta are not excessively desiccated or indurated. When other conditions prevail, the feces are too hard and the bowel does not pass excreta in due time because the serum which should dilute the excrement stagnates in the lungs and thorax. Also, in the early morning sweat bursts forth when the arterial blood is as yet diluted with much serum, because by the help of systole it is extruded through relaxed pores at the time of very quiet sleep.[220] Thus far it is not clear what is truly the basis by which when thin clear urine pours forth in large amounts it is possible to predict both an asthmatic attack and dropsy. Willis[221] in his *De Urinis*, chap. 4, p. 185, rejects curdling of blood and nerve fluid as a cause. He says,

I have known certain women of delicate and very fine texture who occasionally felt unwell for several days and [at such times] usually voided daily huge amounts (more than twice the amount of liquid ingested) of watery urine, thin and without solids or sediment. At this time they

[214] Christophorus Guarinonius, *Consilia Medicinalia* (Venice, 1610), consilium 349, pp. 357–358.

[215] Apparently this refers to Steno's *De Musculis et Glandulis* (Leyden, 1683), but I have been unable to find the relevant passage.

[216] J. C. Brunner, "De Experimento Circa Motum Musculorum," *Miscellanea Curiosa sive Ephemeridum Medico-Physicarum Germanicarum Academiae Caesareo-Leopoldinae Naturae Curiosorum*, Decuriae III, Annus Quintus et Sextus, obs. 293, pp. 659–661 (Frankfurt and Leipzig, 1700),

[217] Riverius, *op. cit.* (footnote 4), book 7, chap. 5, p. 460.

[218] Johannes Nicholas Pechlin, *Observationum Physico-Medicarum Libri Tres* (Hamburg, 1691), book 3, obs. 39, pp. 517 ff.

[219] Saxonia, *op. cit.* (footnote 90), book 1, chap. 1, p. 152.

[220] The authors apparently mean that sweating occurs in the early hours of the morning because serum has not yet been extruded via the pores. In their opinion such extrusion should normally occur after some hours of tranquil sleep.

[221] Thomas Willis, *De Urinis*. In his *Opera Omnia* (Amsterdam, 1682), pp. 152–172 (see esp. p. 158).

would complain of faintness, difficult respiration, and inability to move. I suspect that in this case the blood and the nerve fluid become excessively acid through loss of salt and the occurrence of menstruation; for that reason [those fluids] become susceptible to partial resolution in mixture and to excessive conversion into serosity.

Assuredly if the situation were altogether as Willis states, although there is no lack of doubt, yet in the case that we are discussing, it is highly improbable that acidity of the blood, if it were present to the maximum extent, would immediately threaten an asthmatic attack and dropsy. Rather we are of the opinion that an abundance of thin clear urine evidences spasmodic contraction of viscera in those who subsequently lapse into dropsy. Moreover, contraction of this kind, if it occurs somewhat frequently, is usually the prolific source of obstructions and of the evils which develop from them, and it would not even be so very incongruous to predict asthma and dropsy from visceral contractions of this kind. In addition it is not necessary for us to explain why, when dropsy increases, the urine is scantier and of darker color and deposits various sediments, since no one can be unaware that urine of this kind provides a sign of serum effused in the chest, and of viscera in bad condition, and of increased fever.

After miseries suffered for a long time our dropsical patients must leave this world. Some, whose lungs are compressed by an excessive quantity of serum, die as if suffocated, all respiration ceasing with [the cessation of] life. Other dropsical patients, who have serum effused into the brain or accumulated gradually among the convolutions, die in convulsions or apoplexy. For in this way kindling-wood is furnished to those diseases which snatch away life. It is likely that serum stagnating in the brain either erodes the pia mater by its acrimony or bursts it by its quantity and, flowing down into the base of the brain, corrupts by its stagnation the medulla oblongata and the nerves which originate there, or immediately irritates by its sharpness. When this happens, convulsions, apoplexy, and other evils must follow. The diversity of fluids which are found in the bodies of dropsical persons after death is due to the different constitutions of the bodies and of the fluids within them, and also to the length of time [those fluids] have stagnated in the chest. And since in previous [passages] we have already touched on the diseases of the viscera, we may now rapidly advance to the treatment of the disease.

Chapter III

In Which the Treatment of Dropsy of the Chest is Given

Summary

1. Serous accumulation collected in the lungs and chest must first be evacuated, and assuredly by external remedies.

2. How [serous accumulation can be relieved] by internal remedies, and first by purgatives.
3. By diuretics.
4. By diaphoretics.
5. By pectoral remedies.
6. How maladies of the fluids and viscera should be corrected.
7. By what method the symptoms of this disease should be counteracted.
8. How the power of respiration should be taken care of.
9. This disease is almost incurable.

1. In treatment all considerations should be directed to (1) how the serous accumulation in the lungs and chest may be evacuated by any method whatsoever. (2) Zealous precautions should be taken that a new accumulation does not subsequently form. This occurs especially when diseases of the viscera are removed and every cause of cachexia is turned away by the protection of our art.

Both conditions are very difficult to achieve. Riverius,[222] in the work already cited, characterizes the disease as very serious and very refractory to treatment. "In those," says he,

who suffer from it, the natural heat is altogether weak and the natural forces languish because of some serious disease of the viscera. Hence it happens that although the collected fluid is evacuated by suitable remedies, which is difficult, afflux of new material occurs; by this the disease is not only fostered but grows daily worse, so that at last the body falls into a dropsical ascites.

Likewise Rodericus à Fonseca[223] emphatically says on page 376 that "this disease cannot be cured and that the services of art and nature do nothing." And Petrus Salius Diversus[224] in his De Affectis Particularibus (On Special Affections) page 247 in the same way doubts "whether the physician can satisfy these indications." Nevertheless he admits that

those whose treatment he undertook he liberated from this disease of the chest for certain periods of time, after he had removed the peccant matter; and he had kept them alive for months and for years, although with very great difficulty.

Moreover there are cases in which this dropsy of ours has been cured. Notable among them is the case of Willis,[225] which is reviewed on page 218 of the work already cited. Therefore patients should not be deserted, or abandoned merely to a prognosis. On the contrary, strenuous efforts should be made in order to satisfy both intentions[226] to the extent of one's ability and to prolong the life of the unfortunate patient for at least a short time.

At the beginning it should be noticed immediately whether some trickle [of hope] flows from surgical

---

[222] Riverius, op. cit. (footnote 4), book 7, chap. 5, p. 460.

[223] Fonseca, op. cit. (footnote 38), consult. 54, 1: p. 197.

[224] Petrus Salius Diversus, De Febre Pestilenti Tractatus, et Curationes Quorundam Particularium Morborum (Harderwijk, 1656), p. 247.

[225] Willis, op. cit. (footnote 45), sect. 1, chap. 13, pp. 229 ff.

[226] The intentions stated at the beginning of chapter III of the present treatise.

sources, by which the water can be removed from the chest. In the *History of the Diseases of Breslau for the Year 1699* [227] we have already explained what help can be hoped for from venesection in ascites; we promise no greater advantage to anyone from this method in dropsy of the chest. Indeed, we predict irreparable harm. This happened about six years ago to a man of high rank in whom, on the advice of an experienced physician, venesection was used quite generously. In a short while he went away to the majority.[228] After the venesection all his symptoms increased, especially the difficulty of respiration. In his *Consultations* Benedictus[229] wisely remarks that "venesection should not be mentioned, since it is altogether inappropriate, both on account of cold humors and on account of atony of the viscera."

Some men recommend paracentesis, others condemn it. Among the latter is Riverius[230] who says on page 256, "I am absolutely unable to approve opening the chest, since I have not seen [this procedure] recalled to use and I have not read in any author that it has given a happy result." Petrus Salius Diversus[231] states, in the book previously cited, that he had not dared to cut into the chest or to approve this being done by others, "because the cure of this disease requires not merely that the material which presently obstructs and fills the lung be removed but also that it be prevented from forming anew." Moreover, "incision [into the chest] can only satisfy the first indication and not the second." From this, Salius Diversus concluded that paracentesis cannot be a sufficient treatment for this disease.

In our own opinion this is not in dispute. The discussion is only about whether paracentesis has a place in dropsy of the chest, even though we grant that it may not be a sufficient remedy. Nor should Diversus have rejected paracentesis completely, inasmuch as evacuants are also not a sufficient remedy, yet our learned Doctor Salius values them highly.

Of greater weight is an argument which others advance. Doubtless water is frequently held not only in the chest but also in the lungs; that which is in the lungs obviously cannot be drained away by cutting into the chest. It is of great importance to us to acknowledge that unless it has been established by undoubted signs that there is water fluctuating in the cavity of the chest, incision should not be done. But some authors do not doubt that, if the presence of water has been disclosed, there might be a place [for thoracentesis], skillfully performed. Among those [who hold this opinion] are Hippocrates, or whoever

is the author of the *Liber de Morbis*; also Sylvius, Willis, and others. Indeed, Sylvius[232] says in his *Praxis*, book I, chapter 50, page 316,

if it is well established that dropsy of the chest is present, I do not see why it should not be permissible to do paracentesis of the chest through a harmless hollow silver needle; assuredly a wound of this kind threatens no danger to the patient.

This opinion is contested by the learned Horn,[233] who says in his *Microtechne* that the procedure is clearly not without danger. But he rightly advises that opening of the chest may be approved finally when nothing is being accomplished by medicines.

Willis[234] in company with Lower performed the same [procedure] successfully on a healthy young man, as can be read on page 216 [of his *Pharmaceutice Rationalis*]. Since this history clearly teaches the manner in which paracentesis should be performed, it seems worthy of being inserted here in full. It is as follows:

After having prepared everything the surgeon applied the cautery between the sixth and seventh vertebrae. The next day he inserted a pipe into an orifice cut into the cavity of the chest. As soon as this had been done, a thick fluid resembling chyle, whitish and almost milky, flowed out. Only about six ounces of this material was removed at the first attempt and a similar amount the next day. On the third day, when a slightly larger amount was allowed to escape, the patient immediately suffered great weakness. He then was feverish for a day or two and felt ill. Therefore it seemed best to stop the drainage of the fluid until he should regain his [humoral] temper and his strength. Subsequently the evacuation of the same material was made each day, sparingly, and. the cavity of the chest was emptied almost completely. Up to the present time he still wears the tube in the orifice, with a stopple. When the tube is opened for the period of a day and a night the fluid emerges almost entirely. Meanwhile the patient, healthy in his digestion, appearance, and vigor, has been walking about outdoors, riding, etc. He has taken little medicine and needed little. After the incision we ordered him to take cordials in moderation, occasional hypnotics, and subsequently a vulnerary decoction twice a day.

Thus Willis wrote. But to us it is apparent, although we make no admonition, that in this incision of the thorax the same precautions should be observed that are ordered in paracentesis in ascites. We have already made a few remarks about this in the clinical history and the subject is more extensively discussed by Heurnius[235] in book 6, aphorism 27, n. 3, Capivaccius[236] in *Practica Medicina* book 3, chapter 19, also

---

[227] *Historia Morborum Qui Annis MDCIC, MDCC, MDCCI Vratislaviae Grassati Sunt*, a Colleg. Acad. Leop. Nat. Curios. Vrat. in Lucem Edita (Breslau and Leipzig, 1706), pp. 124–125.

[228] I.e., he died.

[229] Julius Caesar Benedictus, *Consultationum Medicinalium Opus* (Venice, 1659), consult. 42, p. 184.

[230] Riverius, *op. cit.* (footnote 4), book 7, chap. 5, p. 460.

[231] Salius Diversus, *op. cit.* (footnote 54), p. 246.

[232] Franciscus Sylvius, *Praxeos Medicae Idea Nova*, book 1, chap. 50. In his *Opera Medica* (Amsterdam, 1580), p. 316.

[233] Joannes van Horne, *Microtechne, seu Methodica ad Chirurgiam Introductio* (Leyden, 1668), p. 134.

[234] Willis, *op. cit.* (footnote 45), sect. 1, chap. 13, p. 230.

[235] Joannes Heurnius, *Hippocrates. Aphorismi Graecè et Latinè*, edited by I. Heurnius (Leyden, 1601), book 6, aphorism 27, no. 3, pp. 440–441.

[236] Hieronymus Capivaccius, *Practica Medicina*, book 3, chap. 19. In his *Opera Omnia* (Frankfurt, 1603), p. 735.

Mercatus,[237] Rudius,[238] Hollerius,[239] and our Scholzius[240] in aphorisms 1128 *et seq.* As for the procedure, all the details have been quite accurately set forth by the most experienced surgeon Cornelius Solingen[241] in the *Handgriffen der Wund-Artzney* part 2, chapter 1, p. 175 *et seq.*

But what should be said about issues and vesicants and whether serum stagnating in the [thoracic] cavity can be evacuated by their aid? Mercatus[242] and Rudius[243] distinctly approve. We have often observed the value of vesicatories, carefully applied, to be quite remarkable, not only in the more persistent painful affections such as refractory headache, hemicrania, toothache, and in arthritis which is not yet inveterate, but also in the more dangerous symptoms of acute diseases, convulsions, deliria, and retrocedent exanthemata; but here we do not precisely understand what they can contribute to the main issue, unless perhaps someone should convince himself that by these measures the sero-lymphatic fluid can be turned away from the chest and led off to the external parts. Slower help is to be expected from issues, which otherwise are commendable for their outstanding usefulness after a period of several weeks in affections which recur frequently, such as ophthalmia and ocular inflammations, difficulty of vision and hearing, etc. We cannot at all recommend the seton for efficacy in removing a serous accumulation that has effused into the cavity of the chest, [although] we have applied [this device] successfully on several occasions in quite severe catarrhal affections about the head that have already become partly inveterate.

When dropsy is increasing steadily and the feet swell, scarification certainly has a place. Our colleague Dr. Helwich has applied it on several occasions, and also in the Jesuit whom we have mentioned in chapter I. After a scarification had been made in the left foot and repeated for several days, it is incredible how much serous fluid emerged during several weeks. In the right foot the effort did not succeed as had been hoped, perhaps because the skin at that place was thicker and the fat more abundant, until he had recourse to scarification made with a sweeping motion. Thereupon a large amount of water flowed out but the patient had no relief. Meanwhile he took special care lest gangrene or sphacelus should occur, of which at times there was danger; this happens not rarely, as

Ludovicus Septalius[244] correctly observes in the seventh book of his *Animadversions*, note 56.

In addition, if any benefit is to be obtained from incisions of this kind, the humor must be sufficiently fluid; if it is too gelatinous, incision is made in vain. We know that these scarifications are not approved by all, but we consider it useless to fight against experience, inasmuch as we read that since the times of Hippocrates the operation has been done many times with salutary effect. An operation of this kind is very famous among the Egyptians, and the words of Prosper Alpinus in his *De Medicina Aegyptorum*,[245] book 3, chapter 13, page 102, deserve to be quoted here. "Not rarely," he says,

they treat dropsical persons by incision, drawing out the water. Different men use different incisions for this purpose. Some make three wounds below the umbilicus for a distance of three fingerbreadths toward the direction from which the dropsy has originated. Others scarify the swollen belly with small scarifications, through which the water comes out little by little. Others safely make two incisions above and below the arches of the feet on the inner side and the outer side. Through these [incisions] the water is drained away conveniently and gradually. I have seen several persons cured of extensive dropsy by this kind of section.

On the next page [of the same book] Guilandinus[246] teaches that "this kind of treatment was very well known to the ancient physicians, not only with respect to the two kinds of dropsy[247] but also with respect to watery hernias[248] and all watery swellings."

Moreover, we are of the opinion that puncture can be done, with benefit to the patient, even in swelling of the scrotum; Dr. Helwich recently undertook this in a distinguished personage and Dr. Grassius[249] in a miller. For the fluid emerges in large quantity and although the swelling recurs in a short time, as happened in both patients, it is easily evacuated again if the wound is kept open. At the proper time the wound is easily healed by the application of vulnerary medicaments and balsamic decoctions. Not only did the fluid disappear; likewise the asthma with which the patient was miserably tormented in time subsided. For the removal of water from the body of the Most Serene William III, King of England, Nickholson [*sic*] the English physician recommended various external remedies; as G. Bidloo[250] reports in the

[237] Ludovicus Mercatus, *Libri Duo de Communi et Peculiari Praesidiorum Artis Medicae Indicatione* (Pintiae, 1574), book 1, chap. 15, p. 451.

[238] Eustachius Rudius, *Ars Medica* (Venice, 1608), book 2, p. 89.

[239] Hollerius, *op. cit.* (footnote 201); passage not found.

[240] Laurentius Scholzius, *Aphorismorum Medicinalium* (Breslau, 1589), aphorism 1128, p. 263.

[241] Cornelius Solingen, *Hand-Griffe der Wund-Artzney* (Wittenberg, 1712), part 2, chap. 1, pp. 175–188.

[242] Mercatus, book 1, chap. 15, pp. 448 ff.

[243] Rudius, book 2, p. 89; book 1, p. 191.

[244] Ludovicus Septalius, *Animadversionum et Cautionum Medicarum* (Dordrecht, 1650), book 7, note 56, p. 205.

[245] Prosper Alpinus, *De Medicina Aegyptorum* (Venice, 1591), book 3, chap. 13, pp. 102–104.

[246] Guilandinus is one of the discussants in the dialogue presented in Alpinus' treatise.

[247] Thoracic and abdominal.

[248] Presumably hydrocele.

[249] Possibly Sigismundus Grassius, who collaborated with Conradus Victor Schneider in *Disputatio de vera natura et recta ratione curandae phthiseos conscripta.* (Wittenberg, 1648). See also A. Haller, *Bibliotheca Practicae* (Berne, 1776–1778), 3: p. 339.

[250] G. Bidloo, *Bericht von der letzten Kranckheit und Tode Wilhelm des III, Königs von Gross-Britannien.* Aus dem Holländischen übersetzt (Leipzig, 1703), pp. 104 ff.

Bericht von der letzten Kranckheit und Tode Wilhelmi III, p. 104, no doubt he believed the evacuation could be obtained:[251]

(1) By means of fresh groats, sand, and salt—all these dry and warm.

(2) By a little box, which one can carry with him, made of earth or other material from the mountains.

(3) By incense made from plants, wood, minerals, and other spirituous substances.

(4) By the smoke collected over a hole in the earth in which a fire has been made.

(5) By malt, that is to say when the beer is skimmed off; also by herbs, lignum vitae,[252] all kinds of powder, and liquids, prepared by cooking. And Bidloo adds: "all this can be used safely."

2. From external remedies we must proceed to internal remedies. Among these, purgatives must be mentioned first. Practitioners unanimously recommend them in this disease, although some men advocate certain ones and some advocate others. For even in this there is no single opinion. The learned Martianus prefers manna, which he believes drives out serum that stagnates in the chest. Petrus Salius Diversus[253] advocates two [drugs] which, he proclaims, have been of great usefulness; one is elaterium, the other is the juice of the roots of sambucus. Of the latter he gave as much as an ounce and a half, of the former a maximum of four grains.

Rodericus à Fonseca,[254] p. 377, judges that elaterium is a dangerous drug and should therefore be avoided. He himself advocates two medicaments, which, following Fernel[255] in book VII of *De Methodo Medendi* he considers to be far more efficacious for purging away water, but for the evacuation of serum he praises especially the seeds of the dwarf-elder in doses up to 1½ drachms with sugar and cinnamon. Riverius,[256] p. 256, believes that among the hydragogues which are derived from minerals, the most effective in this disease is mercurius vitae[257] so improved that it evacuates from below only. The purgative hydromel of Willis[258] contains as purgatives cardamom seeds, elder, senna leaves, agaric, mechoacan, and turbith. His pills consist of mercury and resin of jalap. For its remarkable effectiveness Dr. Helwich praises the electuary hydragogue that

Dr. Sylvius[259] describes in book 1, chapter 7, page 170 of his *Praxis*, but up to this time he has never given this medicine in the presence of fever. Indeed he believes that on such occasions all the drastic and very strong evacuants should be far away. Since it is nevertheless advantageous to patients to have their bowels open, he has thus far used lenitives only. Meanwhile he extols with great praise the lenitive electuary of Burrhus, because it has a pleasant taste and opens the bowels very gently by lubrication without any disturbance or intensification of fever. Nevertheless for many reasons he does not hesitate to exhibit another medicament that has become known by the name of perpetual balsam; it is powerful through its extraordinary property of relieving the obstruction of viscera and of protecting them from putrefaction. As has been discovered on several occasions, it exerts these effects quite obviously in those whose ordinary drink is beer. Lister's sacred tincture, made from hiera picra[260] and cochineal, which he mentions in his consultation on the Most Serene King William [III of England] also deserves mention among the more choice medicaments. However his pills[261] of hiera picra one scruple; extractum rudii four grains; licorice juice, four grains; solution of rose water, one scruple per dose; are nauseating because of their excessive size and their taste. Nevertheless our Sennert[262] in book II, part 2, chapter 20 of *Medicina Practica* has wisely advised that "the [fluid] matter should be drained away gradually and that purgative drugs should be repeated." For if in dropsical patients the water flows out all at once, they generally die, as Hippocrates[263] says in the *Aphorisms*, parag. 27, sect. 6. And even if perchance this does not happen, if the purgative is given too strongly, there certainly occurs what Riverius[264] observed, [namely] "that the fluids are strongly disturbed, whence a great suffocation befalls the patient and suddenly carries him away. Therefore," he says,

the thing should be done carefully and medicines should be used in smaller doses and on repeated occasions, and should be mixed with the more powerful aperients and diuretics, so that at the same time the passages are opened and a portion of the serous matter is led to the pathways of the urine.

3. In the treatment of dropsy of the chest diuretics follow purgatives. From diuretics the most glorious Emperor Maximilian II derived much advantage.

---

[251] The Breslau text gives the five numbered items in German.

[252] Guaiac.

[253] Salius Diversus, *op. cit.* (footnote 54), p. 247.

[254] Fonseca, *op. cit.* (footnote 38), p. 198.

[255] Joannes Fernelius, *Therapeutices Universalis seu Medendi Rationis Libri Septem* (Frankfurt, 1593), book 7, pp. 355–356.

[256] Riverius, *op. cit.* (footnote 4), book 7, chap. 5, p. 461.

[257] According to Lüdy, *Alchemistische und Chemische Zeichen* (Stuttgart, 1913), p. 52, mercurius vitae is Brechpulver, a precipitate of antimony oxychloride.

[258] Willis, *op. cit.* (footnote 45), sect. 1, chap. 13, p. 234.

[259] Franciscus Sylvius, *Praxeos Medicae Idea Nova*, book 1, chap. 8, p. 170. In his *Opera Medica* (Amsterdam, 1580).

[260] A cathartic powder made of aloes and canella bark. *Webster's New Internat. Dict.* (second ed., unabridged, Springfield, 1964), p. 1176.

[261] G. Bidloo, *Bericht von der letzten Kranchkheit und Tode Wilhelm des III, Königs von Gross-Britannien* (Leipzig, 1703), p. 92.

[262] Daniel Sennert, *Medicina Practica* (Leyden, 1628–1629), book 2, part 2, chap. 20, p. 294.

[263] Kühn III. 753.

[264] Riverius, *op. cit.* (footnote 4), book 5, chap. 5, p. 461.

When he had suffered from dropsy of the chest with palpitation of the heart for twenty years, he sometimes voided as much as six pounds in one day. When the flow of matter was impeded, he would suffocate, as Sennert,[265] in the place already cited, reports from Crato.[266]

But the question is, which diuretics have the most important place in this disease. If, as is appropriate, we consider the affected place, you would rightly doubt whether those substances that increase the saltiness of the serum and by that very fact supply the major quantity of the material by which nature is incited to relax the kidneys—that is, saline substances of whatever kind they may be—are wisely prescribed in these circumstances; and whether it is appropriate to prescribe mild acids such as spirits of niter, of salt, or alkaline substances and volatile and especially oily substances, such as spirit of ivory and of tartar, or fixed substances such as salt of genista, etc., or finally medium substances such as nitrolated tartar, regenerated niter, and Sylvius' digestive, etc., since it is notorious how harmful such substances are to those lungs are unhealthy, as is the case in our dropsical patients.

And so those drugs especially will be called into use which loosen the mucoid character of the fluids so that it becomes possible for the thinner part of the serum to separate more easily. Of this class are sharp fatty substances, resinous gums, also the root of vincetoxicum, pimpernel, apium, parsley, radish, calamus, and antiscorbutic plants of every kind. From several of these our Döringius'[267] fluid is made for [the treatment of] pectoral dropsy, as is evident from the description in Sennert.[268] The diuretic water of Willis[269] also owes its origin to vegetable substances.

Julius Caesar Benedictus[270] in consultation 43, p. 189 recommends the terebinth above all others. He says, "I have verified [the value of] the terebinth a thousand times in diseases of the chest." Recently a certain volatile ammoniacal salt has gained repute among us because all its properties are derived from sal ammoniac.

Many physicians favor those drugs which are prepared from insects. There is an ancient tradition extending from the times of Archigenes to our own concerning the virtue of millipedes or bugs,[271] by whatever property they work. The pills of Dr. Willis are put together from all these kinds of diuretics in the category last mentioned, for they consist of millipedes, benzoinated flowers of sulphur, powder of the seed of daucus, burdock, and Venetian turpentine.

Pompeius Saccus[272] in Medicina Theorico-Practica, consult. 27, p. 109 recommends the following: prepared powder of millipedes, 2 scruples; succinated salt, six grains; flowers, ammoniacal, seven grains; salts of tartar, [one] grain; with the pectoral and diuretic decoction of Willis. But on this subject Lister[273] obviously goes off into contradictions in his consultation on behalf of King William [III of England], in whom, as is well known, the physicians feared dropsy of the chest, for he strongly advises against all the stronger diuretics, both because "they are too acrid and corrosive" and because they "increase thirst," which greatly troubles patients in our disease, and also because "they overheat the lungs." Indeed, in general it cannot be determined what kinds of diuretics should always be given, but intelligent consideration of circumstances will easily show which diuretics may be called into use and which may be harmful to the patient.

When fever is complicated by dropsy, the stronger diuretics should be avoided. In such cases we have used perch stones,[274] raw crabs' eyes, crude tartar, purified niter, emulsions of violet seeds, etc. Moreover, since nephritic attacks not infrequently increase the dropsy, circumspection is necessary in this situation also. At such times, especially when strangury has been persent, we have ordered a few drops of genuine opobalsam with powdered sugar. There is also a place for the stone of the lynx, for Judaicum, etc.

When no fever is present, in the spring season in robust patients we do not object to the juice of the birch fermented with beer, just as it is prepared in England and elsewhere. The juice of the radish, taken in doses up to several ounces, also produces an increased flow of urine. Strawberries and the berries of the ground-cherry[275] infused in rather weak spirit of wine, if they are taken in an appropriate amount, let us say up to an ounce, excite urination sufficiently. Last spring the eminent Dr. Preuss[276] observed in a certain woman an excellent effect from the essence of ammoniacal gum and the serum of goats' milk; there

[265] Sennert, book 2, part 2, chap. 20, pp. 295.

[266] See above, footnote 40.

[267] Michaelus D. Döringius (d. 1644) of Breslau, relation and correspondent of Daniel Sennert.

[268] Sennert, book 2, part 2, chap. 20, p. 295.

[269] Willis, op. cit. (footnote 45), sect. 1, chap. 13, p. 234.

[270] Julius Caesar Benedictus, Consultationum Medicinalium Opus (Venice, 1659), consult, 43, p. 189.

[271] Assellorum. Nowadays the term Asellidae is used for a family of chiefly fresh-water isopod crustaceans. Some forms, such as the pill bugs and sow bugs, are terrestrial. Webster's New Internat. Dict. (second ed., Springfield, Mass., 1946), pp. 161 and 1318.

[272] Saccus, op. cit. (footnote 65), p. 109; Saccus recommends that salts of tartar be used in the amount of five grains.

[273] G. Bidloo, Bericht von der letzten Kranckheit und Tode Wilhelm des III., Königs von Gross-Britannien (Leipzig, 1703), pp. 89 ff.

[274] Schröder, Pharmacopoeia Medico-Chymica (Ulm, 1649–1650), book 5, p. 331 s.v. percus, perca, says: lapides in capite reperti, juxta spinae dorsi initium.

[275] Physalis alkekengi.

[276] Maximilian Preuss (1652–1721), Physikus of Fraustadt in Poland, later Oberphysikus of Breslau. J. Graetzer, Lebensbilder hervorragender schlesischer Aerzte. (Breslau, 1889), p. 209.

was a remarkable increase in urination and well-being in [her case of] dropsy of the chest and feet; both of the latter conditions, together with the concomitant symptoms admirably ceased and disappeared as a result. Indeed we judge that these and other substances can be used justifiably, in accordance with varied circumstances, when the urine is very thin and scanty. Nor should the affair be managed abruptly, but moderate and continued use is necessary. Laxatives should be given first and also intercurrently; without them the use of diuretics is never safe. Indeed it is necessary that the mass of the fluids first be purged of cruder and thicker sediments lest perchance these pollutions be thrown upon the kidneys and, through diuretics, impinge upon dilated pores; in this way obstruction of the kidneys, suppression of urine, and other evils may arise. Moreover we remember that we have occasionally seen, because diuretics had been used unwisely, that they not only caused great disturbances of the fluids but also produced asthma and the danger of suffocation.

4. Further, diaphoretics also are helpful to our dropsical patients since their bodies abound in serous and vaporous impurities. This is especially the case when the external condition lends itself to perspiration and the very nature [of the patient], as often happens, inclines to sweating, while the patients are still in the more vigorous age. Moreover, to the blood, which in these patients is viscid, diaphoretics contribute fluidity and thinness, and they break up the stickiness of the lymph and open up obstructions. Sylvius[277] has great trust in these remedies and from their immense number he chooses many theriac waters prepared with spirits of wine, decoctions of guaiac wood, juniper, sassafras, royal china root, sarsaparilla, butterbur, etc., scordium leaves, carduus benedictus, carduus mariae, scabiosa, yew, poppy flowers, elder, camomile and millet seeds. Indeed he is of the opinion

that broken lymphatic vessels, after they have been freed by praiseworthy medicines, become united spontaneously, just as I have seen happen in bloodvessels when the proper nutriment of one or other part [of the body] is endowed with the power of adhesiveness because it is more or less sticky and glutinous.

Benedictus[278] in consultation 42, page 184, recommends the decoction of china root with some portion of sassafras wood also for the very reason "it restores tone to the viscera." Hence Willis[279] on page 218 [of the treatise already mentioned] advises that instead of his ordinary drink the patient take the following: sarsaparilla root 6 ounces; china root 4

ounces; white sandalwood and citron, six drachms each; shavings of ivory and hartshorn, three drachms each; aromatic calamine root, half an ounce; seeded raisins, half a pound; licorice root, three drachms; infused according to rule and cooked in 12 lb. of fountain water and strained to six fluid ounces.

Into decoctions of this kind Dr. Saccus[280]—see his consultation 28, page 113 of the book already cited—mixes other substances, such as fumaria, eupatorium, carduus benedictus, arum root, hirundinaria, valerian, etc. But in administering these sudorifics it is necessary to go carefully because of difficulty of respiration; on account of this, Fonseca,[281] on page 378 of the treatise already cited, gives the opinion that "sudorific substances are hard to give." These substances and others of the kind have their place especially when, as usually happens, there is itching of the skin, or excoriations of some kind are present. In this case, according to the opinion of many, it is proper to give the bones of serpents and vipers or even their entire bodies (except for the skin), after discarding all the viscera except the liver. When fever is complicated by dropsy, more than other kinds of medicaments, the sudorifics, carefully selected and given repeatedly, have their use and it is an important one. In these circumstances we are accustomed to give in the morning hours an electuary mixed extemporaneously and made from inspissated juice of sambucus boiled with crabs' eyes, salts of carduus benedictus, and any kind of syrup. Especially at that time, coction being complete, nature has leisure for the separation of residues and the elimination of noxious substances from the body. Indeed we have always been unanimously attentive to moderation in sweating—at other times it does not easily occur in our disease—and have taken pains that the danger of suffocation should not be created and the [bodily] forces should not be depressed excessively. In order to prevent this, subacid analeptics are given during the perspiration if cough, for example, is absent. The loss of strength is less to be feared when the sweat is followed by quiet sleep or by a degree of bodily repose and, what rarely happens, by tranquillity of mind. We have often observed also that the sweats of our dropsical patients are almost uniquely limited; they often burst forth on the chest and head, and very rarely on the limbs. Nevertheless it is not to be denied that these diaphoretics are useless for evacuating water from the cavity of the chest; hence you will hardly read in the older authors that they are recommended for this purpose. Certainly Hippocrates greatly recommended them in fevers, as the distinguished Leclerc[282] observed in book 3, page 1, chapter 21, and therefore they deserve rather to be listed

[277] Franciscus Sylvius, *Praxeos Medicae Idea Nova*, book 1, chap. 50, pp. 314–316. In his *Opera Medica* (Amsterdam, 1680), pp. 314–316.
[278] Julius Caesar Benedictus, *Consultationum Medicinalium Opus* (Venice, 1659), consult. 42, p. 184.
[279] Willis, *op. cit.* (footnote 45), sect. 1, chap. 13, p. 235.

[280] Saccus, *op. cit.* (footnote 65), p. 113.
[281] Fonseca, *op. cit.* (footnote 38), p. 198.
[282] Daniel Le Clerc, *Histoire de la Médecine* (Amsterdam, 1702), part 1, book 3, chap. 21, pp. 199–200.

among those drugs which forestall the cause from producing dropsy.

5. Do pectoral drugs have any place at all in dropsy of the chest? Many [physicians], including the most learned Christ[ianus] Joh[annes] Langius[283] of Leipzig, recommend them. And of course if the lungs are distended by sticky serum and become swollen, perhaps pectoral drugs given carefully will do no harm. But certainly it will be hard for you to understand how they can exert their effect if water moves about in the cavity of the chest, unless you are willing to believe that the lungs on their surface are perforated like a sponge and absorb water and send it off to the trachea to be expectorated, a strong movement of the diaphragm occurring during cough, and by this means whatever substances nature feels to be harmful are pushed forcibly upward. For this purpose the same substances are also recommended that are usually prescribed in empyema of the chest, such as scabiosa, coltsfoot, hyssop, veronica, horehound, lungwort, betony, Venus's hair [adianthus],[284] etc. However, for these to be given justifiably it is necessary that cough be present, since unless nature, as the cough indicates, bestirs itself to eliminate via the lungs the material contained in the chest, it will be altogether useless for us to prescribe expectorants. Up to the present time in prescribing expectorants in this disease we have not gone to excess, since we support the opinion that such drugs have no place unless there are definite indications that mucous matter is sticking about the bronchi and trachea. Even in that case we do not believe that the cautious practitioner can long persist in using them, since expectorants not only eliminate mucous matter in the lungs but also provoke an increased flow of such matter to the lungs; in this respect they work in almost the same way as purgatives, which not only remove dregs from the intestines but also propel feces from the mass of fluids to the intestines. Therefore if any opportunity presents itself for ordering expectorants, the practitioner will not do wrong if he first orders laxatives and the milder cathartics, and does not by excessively prolonged use of expectorants drive viscous substances more profusely toward the chest. It is not necessary to describe at length the method given by Hippocrates in *De Morbis*, book II [285] and in the *De Morbis Internis*[286] on which he relied for purgation in empyema of the lung, since this method is outlined briefly by Clerckius,[287] part 1, book 3, chapter 17. The latter gives this opinion

about it:[288] "Physicians of subsequent centuries did not use it, either because there were no patients who were willing to undergo it or because it was considered useless or impracticable."

6. If by the methods which we have thus far discussed evacuation of the peccant matter were obtained, the treatment would have to be directed to the improvement and correction, as far as possible, of diseases of the fluids, and inflammations, obstructions, and scirrhi of the viscera. For correction of the fluids the following are appropriate; absinth, mint, the lesser centaury, cochlearia, fumitory, nasturtium, carduus benedictus, pimpernel root, scorzonera root, arum, helenium, vincetoxicum, curcuma, rhubarb, ginger, juniper berries, and various drugs prepared from these by pharmaceutical art. Fixed salts also deserve high praise. Among them Arcanum Duplicatum M.[289] is very effective, unless obvious signs of pulmonary damage are present, when the urine is pale. Vitriolated tartar is as powerful as the arcanum. Purified niter itself has great value; absinth salt, when continued appropriately after fevers, is an outstanding drug in dropsy. For correcting viscidity of the lymph and the various ills that arise therefrom, sweet mercury (mercurius dulcis), properly prepared, easily wins out over other drugs. The same medicaments are useful for relieving obstructions of viscera; the more acrid drugs [are suitable] for phlegmatic persons, and the more temperate are for sanguine and choleric persons.

Drugs prepared from animals are devoid of all effect. Examples are the lungs of the fox, or the livers of wolves, calves, geese, chickens, etc., which are considered exceedingly suitable for the lungs, the liver, etc., and some of which are extolled by the physicians themselves. For example, livers [are recommended] by Henricus à Bra[290] on page 90 of his book on simple medicaments for dropsy; Jacob de Dondis[291] of Padua in *Promptuarium Medicinae*, tract. 3, p. 83 *et seq.*; Julius Caesar Claudinus;[292] Schroederus;[293] and others. Nor, by the way, has experience established the virtues that are attributed to toads, by both moderns and ancients, in dropsical diseases. Beyond other remedies we prefer the use

---

[283] Christianus Johannes Langius, *Opera Omnia Medica Theorico-Practica* (Leipzig, 1704), part III, pp. 191 ff.

[284] Johann Jacob Wecker, *Antidotarium* (Basel, 1601), pp. 109 and 484.

[285] Kühn II. 222 ff.

[286] Kühn II. 439 ff.

[287] Daniel Le Clerc, *Histoire de la Médecine* (Amsterdam, 1702), pp. 199–200.

[288] The Breslau authors give the quotation in the original French.

[289] According to J. Schröder's *Pharmacopoeia Medico-Chymica* (Ulm, 1649–1650), book 3, chap. 23, p. 474, arcanum duplicatum is the salt extracted from the caput mortuum or residue of aqua fortis, niter, and vitriol. The significance of the symbol *M* is obscure.

[290] Albrecht Haller (*Bibl. Med. Pract.* 2: p. 267) mentions Henricus a Bra: *Medicamentorum Simplicium et Facile Parabilium ad Icterum et Hydropem Catalogus* (Leyden, 1590 and 1597).

[291] Jacobus Dondus, *Promptuarium Medicinae* (Venice, 1576), tractatus 3, p. 83 *recto*, s.v. Epar.

[292] Julius Caesar Claudinus, *De Ingressu ad Infirmos* (Venice, 1628), p. 158.

[293] J. Schroederus, *Pharmacopoea Medico-Chymica* (Frankfurt, 1677), book 5, pp. 299, 302, 306.

of pills made from the more select extracts, especially in cachexia in either sex accompanied by obstructions of the viscera. But no one can easily determine what should be done in desiccation and dryness of the viscera. Humidifying substances are certainly indicated, but it is not less well established that probably no one has ever been really relieved by their use. If the patient takes, in quantities as great as he wishes, potions of lettuce water, portulacca, mallows, borrago, bugloss, endive, syrup of violets, sweet-smelling fruits, and licorice jujube, you will not see greater benefit from them than from humidifying foods such as scrapings of meat, greens, lettuce, spinach, apples, prunes, cooked raisins, etc., which we greatly prefer to those medicamentous substances. Sydenham's[294] treatment of hectic [fever] by horseback riding, carriage riding, and walking may be added, especially if a strong dry cough is present.

Some men expect great benefit from Venetian soap. This substance scraped with milk and cooked for some time in wine, in imitation of the distinguished Rosinus Lentilius[295] in *Miscellanea Medico-Practica*, part 1, pp. 39, 104, and 176, we have given to patients of this kind, but we well remember that for the most part we did it with slight result. Therefore after a while we stopped using it and in such cases we ordered that herbs, especially the flowers of the lesser daisy, be pounded up and mixed with meat soup. From Wepfer's letter to the eminent Harderus[296] in the *Apiarium*, p. 198 we learned that this method was familiar to him.

7. Having decided these issues in this way, we must discuss in detail the manner in which the more urgent symptoms of the disease should be attacked, namely fever and difficulty of respiration or fear of suffocation. The method on which Saccus,[297] who is praised above, relied for the treatment of complicated fever can be learned from [his] consultation 27, page 109:

To fulfill the first indication (i.e. to decrease febrile effervescence) febrifuges are excellent. For this I advocate the powder of Peruvian bark prepared the French way. If this does not remove the fever, an extract should be prepared from the same bark, gentian root, lesser centaury, and camomile, and salt removed from burned distillation residue should be added to these extracts. Of this, up to one drachm should be given during the two hours before the paroxysm, with half a scruple of diaphoretic antimony and some febrifuge water of Quercetanus or Mynsicht. If the fever is increasing, the diascordium of Fr[acastorius] should be given with water of plantago and vinegar in order to moderate the febrile effervescence. When the

sickness is milder, and alteratives and preparatives are customarily exhibited, deobstruents should be given which usually promote [the flow of] urine, such as salt of vitriolated tartar, one scruple; diaphoretic antimony, fifteen grains; prepared powder of millipedes, one scruple; also a decoction of fennel root, pentaphyllum, grass, iris, and chaerefolium with 10 drops of spirit of niter. The body should be purged lightly with cassia every third day. In this way we attack the febrile matter and also evacuate water, so that the remainder can be absorbed by the lymphatic vessels, etc.

So writes Saccus.

But if, apart from deceit, it is not a fraud for us to express the opinions of our [own] minds, we shall state freely that we do not esteem this treatment. We believe that Peruvian bark, which has strong astringent properties, is extremely harmful in these circumstances. We have learned from varied experience that when it is given, fever of the kind that we are discussing becomes more intense. And every day teaches how much harm it may cause if given unseasonably in true intermittent fevers, of which it may correctly be called the antidote. And if the fever yields as desired, a recurrence is still to be feared as often as the fever is suppressed by this febrifuge immediately after its first onset. For if in this manner the fever "is terminated unaccountably and without favorable signs" and after it has been ended in this way it "for the most part returns," as Celsus[298] correctly teaches in book II, chapter 7, following Hippocrates[299] in the [*Coan*] *Prenotions*:

In those whose fevers cease neither with signs of resolution nor on critical days, a recurrence is to be expected.

Indeed, this is not the place to enter into a hateful disputation on the harmful abuse of this drug. And we shall not be responsible for anyone profaning the diascordium of Fr[acastorius] by empirical use. It is in other respects an excellent remedy in contagious diseases. However, both because of astringents and opium, which enter into its composition, it cannot be given safely in this disease. Considering that these fevers arise especially because there is a morbid condition affecting the viscera, e.g. infarcts,[300] tubercles, scirrhi, broad indurations, etc., by which the blood is precluded from free movement, we have thus far held that they should be treated in no other way than are hectics, and we have scarcely prescribed anything but drugs which remove obstructions, cut into [morbid areas], and resolve them. In the *Consultations* of Saccus it is pleasing that the author recommends the diuretic method; what is not obtained by this means you will scarcely accomplish by any other, although

[294] Thomas Sydenham, *Opera Omnia*, ed. by G. A. Greenhill, (London, 1844), p. 198 (*Observationum Medicarum*, sect. 4, chap. 7) and p. 430 (*De Podagra et Hydrope*, 1, 39).

[295] Rosinus Lentilius, *Miscellaneo Medico-Practica* (Ulm, 1698), part 1, pp. 39, 104, 176.

[296] J. Harderus, *Apiarium* (Basle, 1687), p. 198. Wepfer's letter is dated September 2, 1679.

[297] Pompeius Saccus, *op. cit.* (footnote 65), p. 109.

[298] Celsus II. 7. 9.

[299] This passage occurs in the Hippocratic *Liber Praenotionum*, Kühn I. 116. A somewhat similar statement is found in the *Coacae Praenotiones*, Kühn I. 244.

[300] Not the same as the infarct as understood today; signifies *stuffing* or *engorgement*.

acrid diuretics are to be strictly banned in this condition.

If the complicated fever is a little more aggressive and vehement, it implies the presence of great inflammation, and usually ends its deadly course in a precipitous manner. We have long pondered whether the decoction of guaiac, which Freitagius[301] so strongly recommends in hectic fever, can be given when signs of internal ulceration are present. Danger may arise in moister temperatures and also in those individuals who were formerly infected with venereal taints. In the latter, even in those who are much wasted, it is effective to a degree scarcely credible by the inexperienced, if only the drug is prepared and administered by the method of Arcaeus.[302]

8. There is much discussion about what the physician should do when the respiratory difficulty increases to the degree that fear and danger of suffocation urgently threaten, when the patients and bystanders tremble, and the patient stands at the threshold of death, as can easily be inferred from the pallor of the face and the speed and irregularity of the pulse, the coldness of the extremities, etc. This affection spurns the more inactive drugs; therefore volatile substances doubtless must be given. Since we have often observed that something of a convulsive [character] occurs at the same time, we have selected medicaments which act reliably against both conditions; [thus] we have whitewashed two walls at one time. There is available in our shops a spirit called the bezoar of Dr. Bussius. We have in mind that it has relieved patients; forty drops are given hourly. Sometimes we have also carried on the battle by means of antispasmodic potions, carminatives, and diuretics. We have occasionally been successful with a potion of water of linden flowers, peony, parsley, camomile, ammoniacal spirit c.s.[303] and syrup of dialthea. We have also taken care to have enemas given and we have also ordered liniments made from antispasmodics to be applied. On some occasions appreciable benefit has been obtained from a mixture of spermaceti, oil of sweet almonds, and succinated liquor of hartshorn prepared on the fire with persistent stirring. It dissolves without obvious sediment; but if by chance something is precipitated toward the end [of the procedure], it is so little that it is negligible. When Helmont[304] saw this he construed this kind of asthma as "a paroxysmal [condition] of the lung" and in his treatise De Asthmate et Tussi, sect. 29, he contended that it comes "from poison which by its property affects the lung, just as cantharis affects the organs."

Dr. Helwich learned that tobacco smoke contributes something toward preventing these attacks of suffocation, as was shown by a number of striking examples, to be recounted elsewhere. By what property it accomplishes this, no one can easily explain, even though no one today is ignorant of the fact that tobacco is powerful through sharp oily and salty components. It opens the pores and orifices of ducts, constricts their fibrils, draws out juices from their sources, dissolves and cuts the particles of the blood, and makes viscous substances fluid. For even if these things are true, it is nevertheless not yet established how this aperient and incisive force is able to remove an impending attack of asthma, unless perchance someone would wish to suspect that tobacco exerts this effect by anodyne sulphur.

Wepfer could not quiet an asthmatic paroxysm more rapidly than by repose, with his arms spread out like wings and extended upon an elevated resting-place.[305] At the present time we have under observation a person who insists that [his] asthma is greatly lessened when he inclines his head and strikes his chest somewhat strongly against the table[306] and in this position does some writing.

9. However much we have thus far reviewed the various treatments with which this disease can and should be fought, nevertheless, for the sake of our integrity we believe we should not conceal the fact that often the disease is so rebellious that not only are the patients not cured but their symptoms are not even alleviated. We believe that in this case the patients should be medicated sparingly. Indeed, we believe that physicians would not be doing anything contrary to Christian conduct if for a time they abstained entirely from giving medicine. In this connection Johann Jacob Wepfer, a physician of great repute and perfect experience whom we have often mentioned, shines brilliantly by his example, [as shown] in his own body. In the beginning, as Brunner[307] testifies, on page 161 of the work already cited,

he tried various remedies, but cautiously and wisely. He used aperient diuretics. When he noticed that these troubled his bladder he clung only to the use of gelatin of hartshorn all the time, until by careful attention to drugs he had found out that they were worthless. He took pains only with diet, of which he had always been a most exact observer. With this he was so successful that, beyond expectation, although he did not destroy the enemy, he prevented him from completely occupying the citadel of life for a year or two.

Reminded by his example, physicians will most zealously recommend a very exact diet to their

[301] Probably Johannes Freitagius (1581–1641), whose writings include several works on drugs.

[302] Franciscus Arcaeus, Zwey Chirurgische Bucher. (Nurenberg, 1674), pp. 159 ff.

[303] The meaning of c.s. is obscure.

[304] Joannes Baptista Helmont, Asthma et Tussis. In his Opera Omnia (Frankfurt, 1717), p. 347, §§ 29–30. Helmont saw a similarity between asthma and epilepsy.

[305] Brunner, op. cit. (footnote 39), p. 160.

[306] Pericardial effusion?

[307] Brunner, op. cit. (footnote 39), p. 161.

patients in this disease, bearing in mind, as if it were an oracle, the statement of Lucas Tozzius,[308] on page 311 of the work previously cited: "If there is ever to be any alleviation for this disease, certainly it can be expected only from a most exact diet in which attenuating and drying food is strictly prescribed."

Indeed, this is not enough, but the patients should eat even this kind of food most sparingly and, after the advice of Petrus Salius Diversus,[309] given on page 248 of the work already cited, "should take undiluted wine in very small amounts [only]."

Since great importance is attributed to air in all diseases of the chest and lung, all are agreed that dry pure air should be chosen, free from all contamination. It is known to us that in diseases of the chest the famous Dr. Stahl successfully prescribes inhalation of smoke and vapor of antimony. It is for the future to discover whether this method can be applied usefully in our dropsy.

Fear and terror are extremely injurious to our dropsical patients, and have recently excited great febrile disturbance in the body of a person who had dropsy. These waves of commotion subsided with great distress. The patient was kept alive with almost the same difficulty as Johannes de Pictavia. This man, as Thuanus[310] relates in the third book of his history, was condemned to death. When he was being led to execution, he fell into such an acute fever due to fear, that when pardon was granted by King Francis I out of gratitude to his daughter, who had earned the goodwill of many noblemen by her beauty, the man could hardly be restored to reason and health. From this incident the expression Sanvalerian fever[311] became proverbial among the French.

Finally, efforts should be made to procure appropriate daily evacuations of the bowels. Sleep also should be regulated.

THE END.

GLORY BE TO GOD.

---

[308] Tozzius, *op. cit.* (footnote 101), p. 238.

[309] Diversus, *op. cit.* (footnote 54), p. 248.

[310] J. A. Thuanus, *Historiarum Sui Temporis* (London, 1733) 1: p. 108.

[311] According to Thuanus (*op. cit.*, p. 108) the defendant was named Joannes Pictaviensis Sanvalerius.

INDEX

www.ingramcontent.com/pod-product-compliance
Lightning Source LLC
Chambersburg PA
CBHW081333190326
41458CB00018B/5977

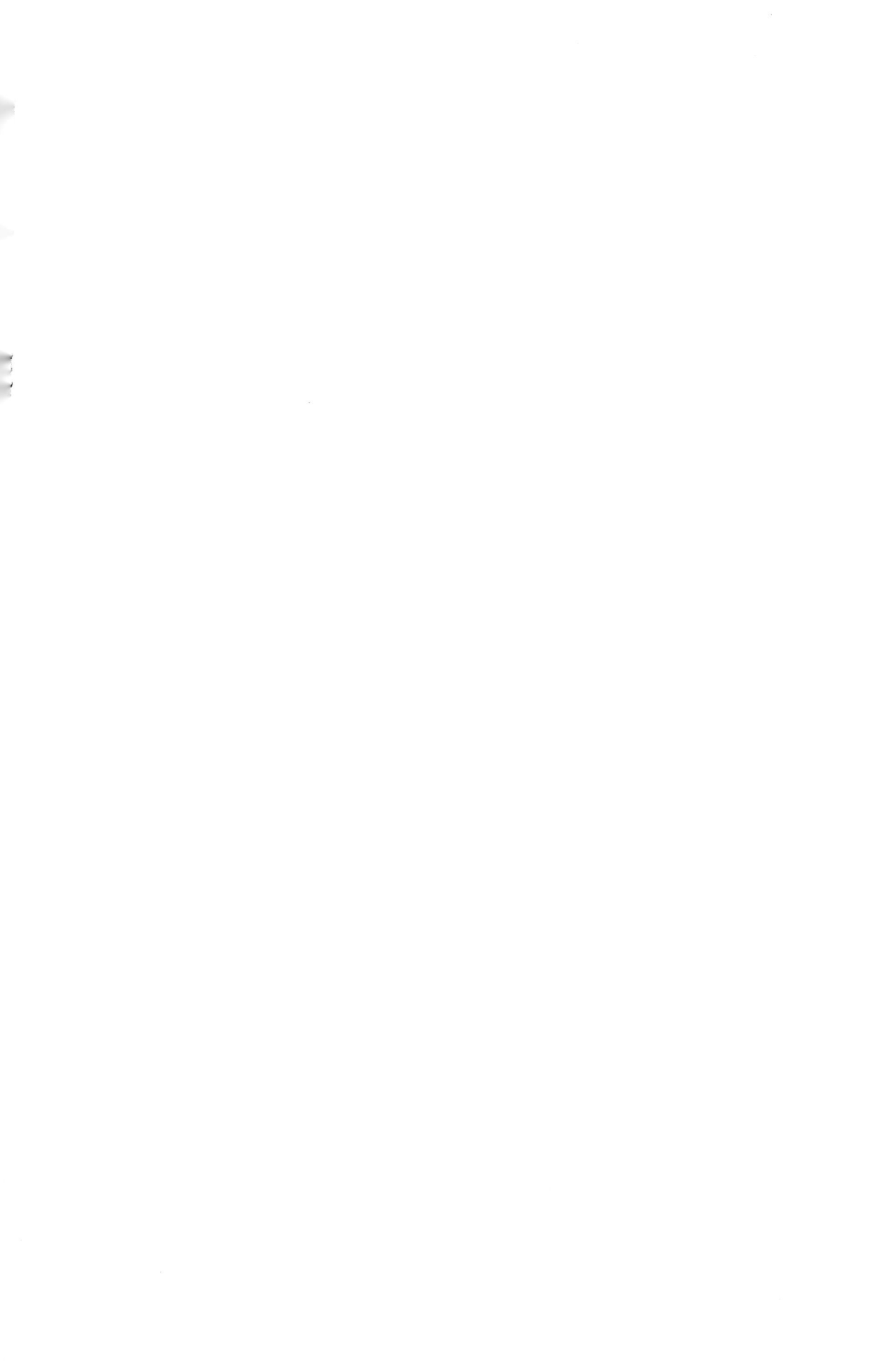